SPIRITUAL PSYCHIATRIES

Mental Health Practices in India and UK

Natalie Tobert PhD

SPIRITUAL PSYCHIATRIES

The author's vision is to explore whether religious and spiritual strategies, to treat mental well being in India, are transferable to services provided in western countries.

The book offers cultural ways of understanding the human self, and presents both mundane explanations for mental ill health, and esoteric theories of illness causation. It explores religious and spiritual treatment strategies, alongside subtle healing. It highlights the Eurocentric management of Indian curricula for psychiatry, psychology and philosophy.

The author suggests Indian principles are relevant to the management of multicultural global mental health care, and offers recommendations for those working with new migrant and refugee ethnic minority populations. The aspiration is that principles around cultural understanding are considered, and then influence medical healthcare education and practice.

SPIRITUAL PSYCHIATRIES

Mental Health Practices in India and UK

Dr Natalie Tobert

United Kingdom 2014

First published by Aethos
http://www.aethos.org.uk/
United Kingdom 2014

The information contained in this book is intended to be educational and not for
diagnosis, prescription or treatments of any kind of health disorder whatsoever.
This information should not replace consultations with a competent health care
professional. The content of this book is intended to be used as an adjunct to
a rational and responsible health care programme prescribed by a health care
practitioner. The author and publisher are in no way liable for any misuse of the
material.

ISBN-13: 978-1494962258

ISBN-10: 149496225X

In memory of Nasreen: we met so briefly

PRAISE FOR SPIRITUAL PSYCHIATRIES

Dr Tobert is to be congratulated on this fascinating exploration of India's healing traditions for psychological illness. Intensive interviews and ethnographic research with certain psychiatrists show a great openness to non-western practices: herbal medicine, astrology, and spiritual healing, which they either directly combine with bio-medicine, or to which they have ready recourse.

Her obvious enthusiasm shines through, and she ends with a short section arguing that these traditions can provide a useful and empathetic adjunct for medical health care for members of the South Asian Diaspora in Britain. Throughout she argues that any sort of therapy has to be meaningful to the people concerned: it has to make sense in their own terms, and not merely be some professional practice imposed upon them.

Roland Littlewood, Professor of Anthropology and Psychiatry, University College London, and Fellow of the Royal College of Psychiatrists.

Western psychiatry and psychology reflect both particular views of the human condition inherent in western culture, and the cultural domination of India during colonialism. The author, Natalie Tobert went out to India and studied how (western-trained) psychiatrists collaborated with indigenous healers to help people with what she terms 'Spiritual Psychiatries'. She describes some of these practices and then explores ways in which knowledge about what happens in India can be used to inform mental health systems in UK.

The result is a remarkable work containing information that few people working in mental health have access to. The book is both informative and thought provoking. The observational studies should be of interest to Indian readers and the lessons drawn from them should enable workers in the UK mental health field to improve the services they provide to people from non-western cultural backgrounds.

Suman Fernando, author of: 'Mental Health, Race and Culture'. Former Consultant Psychiatrist, Toronto University gave a 'Lifetime Achievement Award for 'Culture, Race and Mental Health'.

Spiritual Psychiatries is a fascinating and thought-provoking read. Based on anthropological methods, the book richly reflects on how culture, religion and bio-medicine have vied for influence over understanding about mental health difficulties in India. The compelling ideas developed in Spiritual Psychiatries provide important insights into how mental health services can be improved across the globe.

Dr Ross White, Coordinator MSc Global Mental Health Programme, University of Glasgow

❖ ❖ ❖

The Western psychiatric diagnostic culture is under debate. The question is, do we really reduce the suffering and pain of our patients and create well-being? To export our western view does not help us to develop. Maybe we should try it the other way around: with curiosity and an open mind we should look for inspiration in non-Western cultures. Dr Tobert has been doing exactly that for many years. Her book is a must for those of us interested in complementary medicine and psychiatry. Read it!

Bo Ahrenfelt, psychiatrist and psychotherapist, in Sweden

This book illustrates the importance of multicultural awareness and the need to determine appropriate ways of supporting people with mental health problems, by listening and responding to their stories in a culturally sensitive manner. Within Western psychiatry, a reductionist medical model is only one of many possible approaches.

Dr Katherine Darton, Information Officer, National Mental Health Charity.

AUTHOR'S NOTE

This book is a work of non fiction. Individuals and organizations are called by their real names, except where I have used pseudonyms to protect the identity of patients.

My aim is that this book serves to enhance social well being. I wrote it to raise awareness of alternative models of health with front-line medical and health-care staff, social workers employed with multicultural populations, and front line police officers. It is also useful for chaplains and other religious leaders, both within hospitals and in the community. The book supports government visions for seamless healthcare.

CONTENTS

ILLUSTRATIONS

Line Drawings by Graham Reed

ACKNOWLEDGEMENTS

I am grateful to the British Academy, the Society for South Asian Studies, and the Religious Experience Research Centre for funding this project over three seasons. During fieldwork in India, I travelled with various members of SAIIIHR (Sri Aurobindo International Institute for Integral Health and Research) including Dr Basu, Dr Mistry, Dr Mohan, and Dr Pani. They kindly translated for me when required, as did Mrs S.Basu, and Arindam. Dr Basu's kind support was instrumental in this project.

I am very grateful for the help given by Naganathan, head priest of the Sri Murugan temple in East London, who was visiting Tamil Nadu. Thanks are due to Graham Reed for the line drawings and maps, and to Jean-Pierre Ribière who took some of the photos. A huge thank you to all those who allowed themselves to be interviewed: their insights and wisdom made this book possible.

I would like to thank Shahram who read and commented on drafts of the manuscript, and whose support and input were invaluable. Finally, I am grateful to Ravi Patel who gave me encouragement to complete the project. Thank you all.

Dr Natalie Tobert

London, April 2014

FOREWORD

This is a beautiful and highly informative book. In simple language, and with great honesty and transparency, Dr. Tobert takes us on a fascinating tour through a variety of mental health practices in contemporary India, both secular and spiritual. To her credit as an anthropological participant-observer, along the way she shares some of her own subjectivity, which both humanizes the narrative and humbly discloses the limits of her knowledge. In the last part of the book, she takes us from India back to the UK, where the health system faces challenges in caring for a multi-ethnic, multicultural, multi-generational population. Here, she convincingly argues for the importance of educating clinicians about a variety of world views, explanatory models of illness, and cultural practices that lie outside of the standard Western bio-medical model. For only by making a sincere effort to understand people can clinicians actually communicate with patients, and thus forge an effective working alliance.

In the following pages, you will read some remarkable examples of how psychiatry and spirituality can be integrated in both theory and practice. For instance, Dr. Basu's collaboration with a Muslim occultist in Bengal is a new kind of work that is virtually unheard of in Europe or the United States. In part this creative synthesis is due to the ancient genius of Indian culture, which has always fostered spiritual and philosophical syncretism. However, in part it is also due to structural differences between mental health care in India and the West. In India, most care is delivered in a private practice setting. There is little government or private insurance, little regulatory oversight, and both patients and practitioners are allowed to self-select each other as the spirit moves them. This freedom allows for flexibility and creativity, as well as mistakes and failure to standardize quality. For similar reasons, in the United States the most spiritually explicit approaches to treatment are also being conducted in private practice. Though one would like to think of combining the best of both worlds, in real life there are unavoidable trade-offs at every step along the continuum from total creative liberty to perfect regulatory control.

The only real criticism I have of this book is that I disagree with myself. Time, life, and more clinical experience have changed me since the interview with Dr. Tobert documented in this book. Today, my spiritual faith and practice are deeper than 10 years ago, but I am also more realistic about just how difficult it is to help some people and some mental health problems. Our knowledge is limited in every sense, scientifically, socially, and spiritually. There is hope, but we have a lot more evolving to do in order to solve the difficult problems of mental health inherent in the human condition.

Still, this book is a welcome step in the right direction. As Lao-Tzu said, the journey of a thousand miles begins with a single step. Many thanks to Dr. Tobert for taking a courageous step forward.

Michael Miovic, MD
Minneapolis, USA

PART ONE

KOLKATA, OBSERVATIONAL STUDY

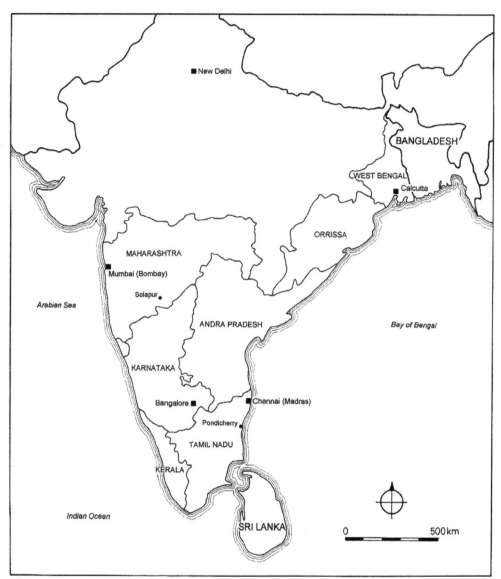

Figure 1 Map of India

Chapter One

INTRODUCTION

Setting the Scene

The psychiatrist's parlour, Pondicherry, South India

My first evening in India: I had just arrived from London to begin a research project on mental health practices. I was there to study bio-medical, religious and spiritual strategies for addressing mental health. I sat in the psychiatrist's front room, with half a dozen of his friends and colleagues.

One Bengali clairvoyant stared at my face and spontaneously started seeing my future: unsolicited.

"You have a blood relative who died between 1995 and 2001."
"No...!".
"She had an active cancer."
"No...!"

SriRam was a small stocky man of great force, in his 30's, with penetrating eyes and a deep black beard. When he needed to concentrate hard, he sniffed the air, flared his nostrils, focused his attention on a grey metal bangle on his wrist, then spoke forcefully of what he saw. When he received 'the force', his eyes bulged. Suddenly a stream of information about me came out, quite unsolicited. The tension in the room increased dramatically. I spoke no Bengali, and he spoke no English. The psychiatrist Dr Basu and his colleagues translated. The 'seeing' carried on relentlessly. The onslaught of words continued with all the subtlety of a ten-ton dumper truck, rolling downhill with no brakes.

SriRam was a seer and astrologer. When the seeing experiences became too much for him, he went psychotic and needed psychiatric drugs to calm him down. The phenomenological experiences were the same, except one was disruptive, the other benevolent. The words 'astrologer', 'clairvoyant' and 'seer' were virtually interchangeable in India.

"There is another female relative, very close to you. She is paralysed and will die very soon. If you don't go back to England quickly then you will not see her incarnate again. Her time of dying is from today. I can see you crying over her body, wearing the same clothes you are wearing today, the same purple salwa khamis. I can see an image of the bed with her form rising vertically from it. She is in peace."

"You will get a shock on 22nd December."

I was already shocked, completely shocked. There were tears in my eyes, and I found it hard to stabilise myself emotionally in front of everyone.

I soon realised SriRam had been speaking first not about a relative, but about my close friend Nasreen, who had died in Oxford, in 1999. Nasreen was an elegant British woman whose family were originally from Kolkata. She had everything: a wonderful family, a luxurious home, bright children, a beautiful figure, a fine mind, and an active cancer. She had always told me she would die young. She was born with the gift of clairvoyance, and would move gently from daily reality to other dimensions at will, with no tools, and no perceptible shift in consciousness. She could do it using her intention alone, remaining in common consensus reality all the while. I first met Dr Basu who was also from Kolkata, at a conference in Oxford, after Nasreen had died, but before she was buried.

I became concerned for my close female relatives. The room was still for a moment. Then the focus of conversation suddenly changed. There was a sense of urgency. The psychiatrist decided my research programme would have to be reconsidered. Originally he said I should leave Pondicherry and go to Kolkata with his colleague at the end of January. Now he said I should go with him straight away in early December. There was a lot of talk about my future need to change the flight. Everyone decided that the oncoming trauma at home would mean I would be called away from Kolkata. I needed to change my travel arrangements so I could fly back to UK quickly. Interviews were set up immediately, and phone calls made to temple priests in Tamil Nadu that I wanted to meet. The response of everyone present was without question that everything the astrologer saw was immanent, happening and veridical. They offered to help me gain enough information to satisfy the organisations that funded my research fieldtrip, before I had to return home.

Several hours later that same evening, a majestic older man arrived at the psychiatrist's home. A member of Sri Aurobindo's ashram, he was tall, a body-builder, hearty with a handlebar moustache, a black skull cap, and long white whiskers. His blue bag hung over his shoulder, and his dog Tito, trotted in and sat down beside him, the fluffiest, whitest, best-brushed dog in Pondicherry. Viswajt was a regular visitor and always came with his dog. He also worked as an astrologer and intuitive, and had for many years offered clairvoyant advice to the doctor. He was in his late 60's, also of Bengali origin. He had been living in Pondicherry for the last 50 years, and had been trained in occultism, supported by the Mother (Mirra Alfassa). Viswajt joined in the conversation, and his eyes twinkled. He summoned me over to talk to him, and started looking at me clairvoyantly, unsolicited. He asked the others to put a chair right in front of him and told me to sit on it. He asked to see my palms.

"Your palms suggest that you are influenced by Saturn and Mars, and you've had problems with depression. These are the hands of an occultist. You too have occult powers, but you must use them or you will get sick. Don't turn them down or turn them off. Your health will be affected if you don't use them. Right now you are not mentally or physically strong enough and should meditate fifteen minutes morning and night, then you'll improve"

Then he then sat on the edge of his chair and said *"I don't want to tell you this in front of everyone"* continuing to do precisely that, *"but your mother is dying."*

A lot of the things he said to the group in Bengali didn't get translated. The room fell silent. Everybody looked concerned. And I was close to tears again. The men there simply took it in, in silence. After that he left the house, riding his moped into the dark night, with the fluffy white pooch standing on the floor of the scooter.

I spent the night awake, inviting everyone's thought forms to dissolve, so they would not make manifest what they were predicting. My previous meetings with clairvoyants in the UK allowed me to understand that their seeing was correct within certain bands of frequency, but different psychics would interpret the same event differently. Furthermore I was also aware that the previous year, exactly twelve months earlier, my mother had been taken into intensive care. I wondered whether they were tuning into that time frame and had got mixed up.

The following day I was told everyone had prayed in the ashram for my mother. Their prayers had been heard and this intervention meant she would no longer die within three weeks. With grace, she died seven years later.

My Research Strategy

My aim in going to India was to make an interdisciplinary study of strategies for addressing mental health: bio-medical, religious and spiritual. To this end I carried out ethnographic fieldwork and collected qualitative data over three seasons. Using an observational snowballing research strategy, I visited surgeries of Dr Basu, a psychiatrist from Kolkata in West Bengal, and interviewed colleagues. I used a cassette recorder to conduct purposive interviews with practitioners and patients.

Dr Basu worked in Kolkata and Pondicherry, and therefore my research was conducted in both these places. In Tamil Nadu, with members of SAIIIHR (Sri Aurobindo International Institute for Integral Health and Research) we travelled either by car or train visiting temples, mosques and churches renowned for their healing environments, in particular visiting those which specialised in treating mental distress.

Recorded here are 40 interviews including 25 mental health patients, two philosophers, one Hindu guru and one priest, one Muslim cleric, and two clairvoyants. The remainder were medical or healthcare practitioners, including three psychiatrists, three physicians who were homoeopaths, and one medical herbalist.

The interviews throw light on the plurality of explanatory models for mental illness, the many theories of illness causation, and the multiplicity of treatments used to alleviate mental distress. I have retained the names of the health care practitioners, and changed the names of the patients and carers.

I should mention that the terms 'mental illness' or 'mental health' are not commonly used in India, however, people are more familiar with the usage of: mental distress, and mental peace, and I have preferred these in the text.

In describing this interdisciplinary research into mental health practices in India, I present a synthesis of threads woven through medical anthropology, religion, culture and psychiatry. The book provides an extensive overview of traditional cultural strategies for mental health and well-being, and includes diverse practitioners: psychiatrists, psychic healers, astrologers and clairvoyants. It offers an in depth study of contemporary cultural strategies and practices for mental well being.

For my fieldwork research I used the discipline of medical anthropology, with the technique of narrative ethnography and rich description, which I used throughout the book. This is an observational study of various syncretic health-seeking strategies in India.

This research offered an opportunity to gain profound insight into the plurality of Indian practices and beliefs about mental health, its aetiology, causal factors; diagnoses and treatments. One of my aims in researching mental health practices in India, was to develop a theoretical framework which could be used to explore cultural models of mental health in Britain, with its multicultural populations.

❖ ❖ ❖

Spiritual Psychiatries

The main aim of psychiatry is to reduce individual human suffering. To do this it maintains therapeutic practices which may also serve as a form of social control. In India the use of a multiplicity of medical, alternative, complementary, religious and/or spiritual strategies to address human suffering is not controversial. It is normal syncretic practice for people to try a plurality of treatments to address their well being. Although these are not named 'psychiatry', they appear to have similar functions to psychiatry[1]. Unlike the west, in India there is not one treatment that is termed 'conventional' and another 'unconventional'.

In the west today there are a number of different organisations which teach about alternative approaches to psychiatric treatment. These include the Royal College of Psychiatry in UK, which offers a CPD module (Continuing Professional Development) in understanding the use of complementary and alternative therapeutic approaches. The module leader writes: *"The use of complementary alternative medicine (CAM) for mental health problems is well documented. In psychiatric patients, estimates of the prevalence of CAM use range from 8% to 57%. Such treatments are either used alternatively (instead of) or complementarily (in addition) to conventional medicine."*[2]

The ways that CAM focuses on wellness rather than illness is illustrated in a reference book edited by Dr Philip Muskin[3]. It includes use of yoga, herbal remedies, and acupuncture. In USA, California, the psychiatrist Dr Lake[4] presents evidence based approaches so that clinicians can make appropriate choices about integrated options for mental health care. Another book explores alternatives beyond psychiatry[5] and the authors start from the assumption that modern psychiatric health care with its focus on pharmaceutical drugs does not work, and leads to disability as patients become chronically ill. They search for alternatives to the medical model of treatment and ask *"Why do we need alternatives? What is wrong with the "care" that mainstream psychiatry provides?"* This question has been addressed by service user groups including those under the umbrella of the UK National Service Users Group[6]. The Citizens Commission on Human Rights (established in 1969) produced a compendium on psychiatry, or rather on anti-psychiatry[7].

In UK, the Critical Psychiatry Network was set up in 1999 for medical students and psychiatrists, to develop a critique of psychiatry. Crossley discusses the resistance to psychiatry that grew up in the later 20th century in the UK[8]. Lake and Spiegel ask for an effort to be made *"to integrate treatments that work into mainstream medicines"*[9]. Their book gives the history and rationale for various types of complementary and alternative treatment. In the US, one website offers a selection of non-drug approaches for mental health, with a directory of alternative mental health practitioners[10]. Service users who were unhappy about their treatment, conducted research at the Mental Health Foundation, and produced a fact sheet on complementary and alternative approaches[11]. They have also run a project on Recovery and Resilience which *"explored the concept and settings of recovery from mental and emotional distress in African, African-Caribbean and South Asian women."*

The World Health Organisation has four priorities in Europe: the availability of high quality information; service users' and carers' empowerment; development of community based services; and improving the state of social care homes[12]. WHO explains that *"much is now known about what works in mental health promotion, prevention, care and treatment. The challenge is now to implement this knowledge."* Its report published in 2010, was a call to all governments to focus their attention on mental health.

In this book, it is my intention, not only to present data from an observational study in India, but also to explore in the final chapters, its relevance for UK populations. I would like to address the gap I have perceived[13] between knowledge obtained from academic research, and explore its relevance for frontline health care training and practice in the UK. For example, I worked in the London Borough of Harrow, which according to the 2001 census had an Asian or Asian British population of 29.6%, (a white population of 58.8%, and a Black population of 6.1%). These figures have changed since the last census[14], perhaps due to British foreign policy and wars in certain counties. Harrow had a white British population of 30.9% in 2011. Locally there were support groups for Asian carers and sufferers of mental distress.[15] In Harrow there was also a pilot project run by Time to Change.

Transcultural psychiatry is now offered at more universities[16], and the topic is also covered in Medical Anthropology degrees[17]. There is a Special Interest group at the Royal College in transcultural psychiatry, whose remit is to support: *"policy and practise to improve the care of socially excluded and marginalised groups where culture is influential in the expression and management of mental distress."* Their aim is *"to ensure cultural competency remains an essential component in the assessment of the clinical competencies of all psychiatrists[18]"*.

There are government programmes that address ethnicity and mental health, which include the Count Me In census[19], and the former Delivering Race Equality[20] programme, in which Community Development workers mediated between patients, carers and mainstream services. A response to those two programmes has been compiled by RAWOrg[21], the Rights and Wellbeing of Racialised Groups. Transcultural approaches are now more a normal part of mainstream practices, however, at the time of writing, people from Black and Asian communities feel there is still some way to go regarding cultural understanding and good practice in mental health care[22],[23].

❖ ❖ ❖

Framework

The book is divided into five sections. The first four present data from fieldwork in India, while the last explores issues around transferability of models of health.

Part One: Kolkata, Psychiatric Clinics
Part Two: Treatment Strategies
Part Three: Explanatory Models for Mental Distress
Part Four: Indian Frameworks of Knowledge
Part Five: Transferable Models

Kolkata, Psychiatric Clinics. The first part presents a descriptive overview of my journey from South India to Kolkata in West Bengal. In Kolkata I observed surgeries of a charismatic psychiatrist, who integrated western pharmacological with Indian spiritual treatments for his patients. He collaborated with Hindu and Muslim seers, sages and healers. I describe the psychiatric surgeries, a locked nursing home, and a clinic of a Muslim Cleric on the Bangladesh borders. The Muslim holy man regularly sent patients to the psychiatrist, after determining whether his clients needed spiritual or psychiatric treatment, or both.

This section ends with an analysis of patient interviews, and theories of illness causation, which result in a plurality of medical, religious and spiritual treatment practices being used concurrently. Some triggers for distress were mundane, whereas other causal factors some were 'supernatural', lying outside a materialist paradigm.

Treatment Strategies. In the second section I describe treatment strategies used for mental wellbeing. As well as the pharmacological treatments given by the psychiatrist, various complementary and alternative remedies were used by practitioners to treat patients with mental illness. Remedies included western pharmacology, homoeopathy, herbal medicine, and flower remedies. During interviews I explore practitioners' understanding of the different healing modalities, and the subtle ways they worked towards a patient's well being. For example, one psychiatrist explained flower remedies were good for healing a patient's deep emotional issues. Others felt several kinds of treatment were required to address a patient's condition including pharmacology and prayer.

Next I investigate religious and spiritual treatment strategies like pilgrimage, then present religious establishments like temples and mosques, used by people to address mental distress, and the spiritual ashrams that people visit in order to find mental peace. These chapters illustrate ways people interface with religious and spiritual establishments for the purpose of alleviating mental ill health. Included are visits to the Mahalingam temple at Tiruvidaimarudur, with rituals undertaken, and at Gunasilum temple and Nagore mosque, both renowned for treating patients with mental distress.

I discovered that if a place 'worked', it became renowned for its healing energy, then people of any faith participated in healing rituals, regardless of their religious affiliation. Spiritual places included the palm leaf oracles of Vaitheeswarankoil; the temple of Sri Vaidhyanatha Swami; Suryanakoil, where the nine planets were propitiated; the cathedral of Vailankanni where Our Lady the Madonna assisted healing; and Rameshwaram where healing rituals honoured the deceased. The chapter offers a preliminary glimpse of ashrams of Sri Aurobindo in Pondicherry, and Sri Ramana Maharshi at Tiruvanamalai, where pilgrims sought peace.

Explanatory Models for Mental Distress. In the third section I explore practitioners' and patients' explanatory models for mental distress, including mundane models like psychological or environmental issues, and esoteric models such as effects of planets, karma, and spirit possession. Explanatory models of understanding included biomedical and psycho-social influences on health, based on post-natal experiences and more spiritual models incorporating transpersonal and subtle experiences. I found that there was not only a plurality of theories for illness causation among patients, but also between different kinds of practitioner (psychiatrist, physician, traditional healer).

I considered explanatory models were important because a person's theories of illness causation directly influenced their health seeking strategies, the diagnosis and the strategies they accepted for treatment. Often patients mentioned mundane triggers for distress first, followed by more occult or supernatural beliefs. Spirit possession was sometimes considered a factor in triggering distress, while reincarnation from a human being in a former existence, was thought to be a factor in physiological disorders originating from birth. Planetary influences were considered important, as was karma, or 'incorrect' behaviour in a previous life, which resulted in mental disturbance in this life. Two people explained to me how a discarnate being was created, and why it caused distress to living humans.

Indian Frameworks of Knowledge. In the fourth section I address issues around Indian frameworks of knowledge, and include a discussion between lecturers of philosophy of psychology, and interviews with members of the medical team at SAIIIHR on the relationship between consciousness and health. I explore different cultural existential paradigms around life and health.

I encountered some dissatisfaction and frustration of two lecturers who were obliged to teach psychology from a western academic framework, while they were aware that India had a long history of many psychologies to relieve mental and emotional distress, which they felt were under acknowledged within academia. The three psychiatrists interviewed claimed western psychiatry embodied the underlying assumption that people with mental health problems were influenced by psycho-social post-natal experiences, but because they worked in India they took account of many different influences on their patients' health.

The following chapter describes some philosophies of consciousness, health and illness causation, prevalent among staff at the Sri Aurobindo ashram. It is based on interviews with physicians, psychiatrists and homoeopaths who form the Medical Team at SAIIIHR (Sri Aurobindo International Institute for Integral Health and Research), and includes comments by the late Dr Bisht, founder of the Institute, and the World Health Organisation's former Director General in Asia. I look at the plurality of existential beliefs about human reality, revealed by patient and practitioner interviews, and explore their influence on responses to mental distress. I explore the proposition that beliefs about the nature of physical existence and consciousness after death influence judgements regarding the diagnosis and treatment of psychosis.

Transferable Models. This last section summarises what was learnt from the research. I discuss ways in which the data may be more useful than its face value, as a collection of interesting academic anecdotes about Indian strategies for mental well being. For example, the London Borough of Harrow, where I work, has the 9th most ethnically diverse population in UK. Of its residents, 69% belong to diverse ethnic groups, one third were born abroad, and 28% were Asian. I explore whether the information I gathered was relevant to today's culturally diverse Britain.

I address the current dilemma in UK, regarding ethnicity and the Government's mental health strategy. I explore what happened with the UK governments Delivering Race Equality agenda, and the new mental health strategy, which mentions equalities, but not specifically race equality. The problem is, in spite of these agendas, detention for BAME (Black and Asian Minority Ethnic) groups under the Mental Health Act is not declining, and these groups are still over represented within psychiatric institutions[24]. There is a concern that data on this is not being published, particularly with regards to those of African Caribbean descent[25]. A systematic review was conducted in 2007[26], and the CEO of Afiya (established to reduce inequalities) has asked for race equality to be put back on the agenda for mental health[27].

In the final chapter I present the culturally specific strategies used in the borough to address the mental health needs of its diverse ethnic groups. I explore the extent to which religious and spiritual practices are taken into consideration; and whether innovative cultural frameworks for understanding mental distress might benefit patients in the west. I discuss whether the procedures and philosophies I learnt about in India are transferable to Harrow, and whether this book is of benefit in today's multicultural society. Finally I present a series of recommendations to explore ways to address inequalities in strategies for mental health.

SUMMARY OF KEY BENEFITS

The book explores two propositions, which are essential for medical and health care practitioners who work in multicultural societies, to gain deeper understanding of their patients' beliefs about the causes of mental illness. These propositions are:

- *A person's theories of illness causation directly influence diagnostic decisions and strategies for seeking and complying with treatment*
- *Concordance of understanding of belief system between practitioner and patient improves the potential for healing.*

This book was written to contribute to our knowledge of existential, religious and spiritual elements which enhance understanding of cultural interpretation of mental health conditions. It is of interest to UK front-line medical and health-care staff with multicultural populations; and to medical and health care practitioners overseas who are aware of alternative theories of mental health causation, but discover these are seldom mentioned in training.

The work may also be useful if offered as a resource within medical and healthcare practitioner-training environments; and as a student source book as part of university medical anthropology courses where this kind of material is widely taught as part of the curriculum. For community mental health teams it is useful as a guide to understanding different cultures' explanatory models for mental distress. It creates awareness of patients' concerns, and would be relevant in training colleges for nurses, care workers and psychiatrists. I hope it will also be useful for chaplains and other religious leaders, whether associated with hospitals or in the community, and for General Practitioners and practicing psychiatrists.

As different spiritual approaches to mental health are currently being put forward in the UK, there is surely scope for further collaboration between bio-medical, religious and spiritual practitioners with, potentially, far reaching beneficial prospects for patients and carers. The current view is that cultural competency is fine (gaining knowledge about cultures), but cultural humility is better (ongoing self reflective asking of questions about the other).

Chapter Two

PSYCHIATRIC SURGERIES

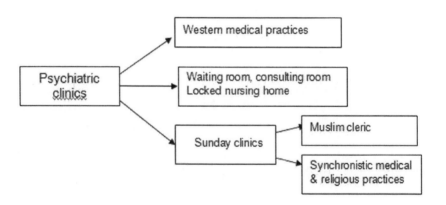

Several days after my friend Nasreen had died, and was not yet buried, but was laid out in a mosque in Stanmore, I travelled from London to attend a conference in Oxford. This was hosted by the British Psychological Society on Consciousness and Experiential Psychology. At lunch time, by chance, I sat next to Dr Soumitra Basu, an Indian psychiatrist from Kolkata (where Nasreen was born). He had given a presentation on Sri Aurobindo and the Psychic Being at the conference.

I explained my intention to undertake medical anthropology fieldwork research in India, and he invited me to join him the following year in Pondicherry. I managed to get grant funding and prepared for the journey. I travelled to Kolkata, where I observed the psychiatrist, and noted his western medical and fusion spiritual therapeutic practices. I visited clinics where he worked in Kolkata, and observed the layout of space. I travelled with him to his Sunday clinics on the Bangladesh borders, and to a locked nursing home.

Journey to Kolkata

My train left Chennai for Howrah station in Kolkata (previously Calcutta). I had a second-class seat with an upper sleeping bunk. We travelled past ruined slum dwellings. All those homes bordering the tracks had been recently torn down, and beside them was a heavy police presence. One row behind, dwellings were still standing. People's possessions were heaped in piles on the ground, among ceramic pots, straw mats and puppy dogs. Those people who had lost their homes appeared resigned: they didn't seem angry. Perhaps they had been offered accommodation elsewhere?

During the afternoon, I found a delightful window seat, where I sat against the wind for four hours in a state of bliss, and watched the world go by. Outside I saw wetlands and dry lands, little ponds by the tracks, birds with long elegant tails that I had never seen before, and flocks of water fowl, with white bodies and long dark feathered necks. There were water buffalo submerged in rivers, and a cow eating from a ceramic jar. In the evening after dark, I climbed back to my upper berth and arranged the sheets on the top bunk.

I thought I slept badly, but the third time I woke up it was morning, and sunrise. Suddenly I transformed from being scared of this two-night journey, and realised I was enjoying myself. Was this not a blessing? Surely it was better than sitting at my office desk? I saw people gathered around the pale flames of a morning fire, working in the fields, building haystacks, and weeding flooded fields of rice lined with coconut palms. I saw field after field of yellow sunflowers, all facing the same way, then seven herons flying across a lake.

Later that morning, three transvestites got on the train: three tall men, with their long black hair tied in buns, embellished with brightly coloured flower garlands. One wore a magnificent burgundy coloured sari and had a long wispy beard. They were begging for money, well not begging, they were demanding money. One put his hand on the book I was reading (Communion with God by Neale Donald Walsh). '*Give me money!*' he said tapping the page of my book. '*Why?*' I asked. '*Give me money!*' he repeated, but his eyes were friendly and smiling. It was the only smiled acknowledgement I had felt so far on that journey, and it filled me with warmth. I seemed to have closed down, become morose, gone within during that journey, and had not made any human contact.

During the day, there were numerous other beggars who boarded the train, crippled and blind, or with shrunken limbs, some singing with drums, some just begging. There was a skinny boy of around eleven, in a loin-cloth. He wore large round glasses and his entire body was coated in white ash. Another man came in with his shrunken leg held up by a stick. One man, who was shaking like an epileptic came in led by a child. And there was a blind singer of modern movie songs who passed through the carriage, led by his companion.

Salespeople walked through the carriage loudly shouting their wares. They sold cigarettes and matches, cucumber and chilli salt, combs and other plastic goods, and chains and padlocks (essential in an open sleeping compartment). There was a pantry car, with *coolies* preparing snacks. Railway personnel walked up and down the carriages, significant in their dark trousers and dark red jackets. They sold tea and coffee from urns in small plastic cups, boxes of samosa, onion *bhajji*, boiled eggs, and individual trays of cooked food covered in tin foil: 'bread omelette', and 'noodles with vegetable'. '*You want the bread omelette?*' '*Yes please, how much?*'

The omelette lay solidly on three chunky potato chips, a plastic sachet of tomato sauce, and two slices of soft buttered bread. It had so many green chillies in it that I had to extract them one by one, and put them out the window. In standard class there was the world outside the window for rubbish dumping, or the corridor between bogeys, which by the end of the journey was strewn with sticky food remains, paper and plastic. In the first class there were rubbish bins in the communal area, and in the super first class, there were plastic pedal bins in the carriage, which were emptied periodically.

I spent two nights on the train, 36 hours sitting, sleeping, waking, eating, and walking short distances at stations. On the last morning, half awake, I opened the train door, and stood for a while with the wind in my hair, watching the landscape go by. Or, was the train going by the landscape? I guess it depended where my centre of perception was. I enjoyed looking out of the window or door, watching water cattle bathing in ponds, the palm trees, the paddy fields, looking into people's homesteads and watching them thresh wheat, cook food, bathe and squat. I saw flashes of people's lives pass swiftly in front of my eyes. In India perhaps it is the journey itself which is grand: one can see things from a train without engaging, without becoming involved. One step removed.

As we arrived in Kolkata, passengers changed their clothes. Those who had worn bright sunny dresses further south, changed into dark clothes, brown jackets, socks and shoes, dark hats and dull coloured scarves. Everyone looked rough and ragged as they prepared to go into the heavy morning Kolkata air. There were hundreds of thousands of people on parallel track commuter trains, wearing hats and shawls, scarves and jumpers. In this cloudy city, heaving with ancient buildings and small streets, it was much colder.

On the platform, the psychiatrist Dr Basu was there waiting with his colleagues. He had ordered a taxi. As I stepped off the train, the clouds parted for a few moments allowing us just one glimpse of the red sun rising, then it disappeared.

Kolkata Streets

The roads to the psychiatrist's home were grid-locked. He lived to the north of the city in the area of Bangur Avenue, about 8 kilometres from the centre. In the streets around his apartment block, roads were roughly surfaced, the main thoroughfares were tarmac, and pavements were non-existent. Slabs of stone covered sewers along the edge of buildings. Electrical wires descended from everywhere, up, down and across the street. The smell of frying fish from the Bay of Bengal permeated the air. I could hear the deep amplified thud of someone's car audio system. There were some parked cars, but very few driving.

Rubbish was ubiquitous, the remains of plastic and paper pecked at by flocks of crows and sparrows. There were motorbikes, cycle rickshaws, women walking in dark woollen shawls, scarves over their heads, and sellers of brushes and brooms. Merchants would walk by or cycle past in the street below, shouting out their wares. There were small retailers and service shops every so often on corners, in amongst all the residential blocks, which were five or six stories high. In the side roads there were stalls for ironing, shoe making, vegetable sellers, and a shop where Internet connection was available. There was a canal a couple of streets away with high-rise blocks on one side and a slum area on the other.

The psychiatrist's apartment was built on the site of an old plot owned by his parents. In the last few years it was raised to the ground and the new block constructed with a purpose built chamber on the ground floor. [The word 'chamber' is used in India to mean the psychiatrist's clinic or surgery, as we might say in the UK.] There were eight apartments in all, and the common areas were well maintained. In each place I visited, I was always introduced to the servants, carpenters and workers, who seemed to stay with families for their whole lives.

Dr Basu's wife was very devout and every day at dusk to honour the transition between day and night with sacred sound, she blew the conch shell. She was a psychologist with particular interest in mental health and criminal behaviour. In the evenings she would sing haunting poems by Tagore. She had an exquisite voice, and her voice rose into the street through the shutters. It was the custom in Bengal for people to entertain each other by hosting singing or poem recitals in their own homes. The couple had kindly invited me to stay with them while I was in Kolkata, to study the way they worked with patients. Dr Basu said he wanted me to interview patients in his Kolkata surgeries, from both urban and rural areas, some priests and Muslim 'molovi' or holy man. He said this one man had a way of judging patients, to determine which were psychiatric cases, and which might be cured by religious rituals.

The Psychiatrist

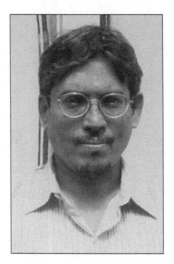

Dr Basu

Dr Basu was born in Kolkata in the 1950's, and as a youth, he had been inspired to study allopathy (or bio-medicine) and psychiatry in particular. He studied medicine at the University of Kolkata from 1973 to 1980, and then did postgraduate work in psychiatry. He had psychiatry practices in West Bengal and in Pondicherry. He undertook co-operative working arrangements with traditional healers, a practice the World Health Organisation encouraged, since it allowed outreach to grass-roots people.

In Pondicherry, he was also part of a medical team who in 1992, established the Sri Aurobindo International Institute for Integral Health and Research (SAIIIHR). Their aim was to explore paradigms of health and psychology from a consciousness perspective. One doctor there explained that although he felt modern bio-medicine had developed unparalleled achievements in fields of specialist research, he considered that various human conditions could not be explained from a mechanistic perspective. He said *"A deeper understanding of the manifestations of ill-health can be found in the visionary philosophies of Sri Aurobindo, who considered that consciousness antedated the manifestation of matter, and was the essence inherent in all reality.'*

Dr Basu held clinics on Tuesdays and Thursdays in his own chamber at Felicity Clinic, Bangur Avenue, and on Saturdays at Serenity Clinic in his in-law's place at Jadubazar. On Sundays he travelled to the predominantly Muslim areas near the Bangladesh border and held clinics at Chowdury, Basirhat and then at Bikshan, Berachampa. He had a consultancy with DumDum Municipal Specialist Hospital, and Sandipani Nursing Home, in Kankurgachi. On surgery days, he worked an exhausting schedule from mid morning right through till 11.00 p.m. barely taking a break to eat lunch. When the doctor was not at work, he was on call. His phone rang all day. Sometimes it continued ringing until 2.00am, and then it began again from 6.00am.

For the first three hours on waking, Dr Basu sat by the phone from 7 to 10am everyday, cross-legged, just waiting for phone calls. There were emergency calls and requests for treatments, which would come through one after the other, after the other. *'Some days families drive long distances, from one to two hundred miles away, just to see me, even though I am not holding a chamber that day. Usually I agree to see people, especially if a relative is psychotic or violent. I offer pharmacological treatments, and in cases where the relatives ask me if in addition they can take intervention of faith healers, I may suggest relatives take the distressed to perform prayers at the local Dakhineshwara temple that was a genuine place. I take this initiative as often village folks fall prey to wrong people when they seek faith healers'.* This was a Kali temple where Sri Ramkrishna, the famous seer and guru of Swami Vivekananda lived and worshipped in Bengal.

Dr Basu also taught each week in the Vidyasagar University, Salt Lake Campus, built on land reclaimed from the marshes in New Kolkata. In the university, the psychiatrist was an inspired teacher. The students listened attentively, sitting in straight rows, behind desks in their small classroom, as he explained to those who specialised in social work and counselling, why the western-influenced training for counselling was not very useful in India. *'One reason is because conventional western teaching assumes counselling sessions are individual, rather than public. Furthermore I feel there is an underlying assumption in western traditions that people are influenced only by post-natal experiences, rather than by past lives, planetary, karmic, or supernatural influences'. 'The western model'*, he said, *'does not fit Indian beliefs about the nature of existence'.* When I conducted research with UK Asian groups, these comments rang in my ears, both regarding the focus on individual counselling, clients' preference for group work, and their beliefs about the nature of distress.

Psychiatric Chambers

The clinic was famous. Dr Basu had never advertised nor had a sign outside. The psychiatrist was well respected locally, known to treat poor people for free. *'I do not take fees, but my patients offer me whatever they feel like. Those who are poor offer nothing and I give them medicines without charge'.* He didn't have a fixed fee: those who could afford it offered him some notes as they left: a hundred or fifty rupees or less, which he stuffed into his trouser pocket without looking. Dr Basu was a sympathetic man who fervently believed in the divine. He got sent patients by holy men, but otherwise he did not appear to use seers regularly to assist with diagnosis, although he did use them to advise on spiritual and religious prayer treatments. He had invited one older astrologer to visit his surgery, to check which of his patients might have spirit possession. But the man said he didn't want to go to the surgery, since he found the energies there difficult.

Patients arrived by the passage outside the apartment block, so they didn't pass through residents' personal space. Outside there was a covered shoe rack, where all footwear was kept neatly. Every patient who attended the surgery was accompanied, by at least one relative, some by both parents, and one girl by both sets of grandparents as well.

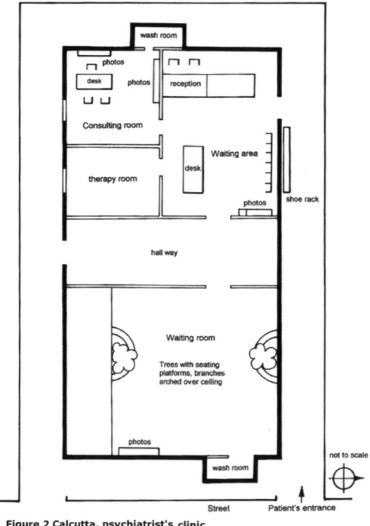

Figure 2 Calcutta, psychiatrist's clinic

Usually the doctor went to his surgery at 10.30 am and didn't go back upstairs to his home until 11.30 pm. He had huge energy during his clinics, often forgetting to eat. He estimated he saw between 90 and a hundred patients each day, and these were all accompanied. That meant around 200 to 250 people came and used the space.

Waiting room. The waiting room of the Bangur Avenue chamber had been decorated to make patients feel comfortable. Builders had constructed two concrete tree trunks, which grew out from the walls, and whose branches spread forming an arch over the ceiling at the centre of the room, with leaves at the top and hanging down. There were seating platforms around the base of the trunk, on which people could and did sit. The floor was of terra-cotta tiles, to look rustic. The walls were covered with rolling hills of green grass, cut out in low relief and covered in green felt, with little palm trees and houses. On one wall there was a red rising sun, with a little light bulb behind to make it glow. On an adjoining wall was a small white temple with two columns at the entrance. Inside were photos of the Mother and Sri Aurobindo, lit up by tiny bulbs. The sky above the miniature temple had crystals attached that caught the light like stars. There were some shelves in the room, which were intended to display artefacts made by the patients.

Dr Basu wanted the waiting room to have a particular atmosphere, since he considered that waiting in itself should be a therapeutic part of the healing process. "*When people come to the chamber, they dress well, even people from lower economic conditions, they wear their best clean clothes when they come, because that is also part of getting well. They want to get well, and people don't mind sitting here for a long time, because sharing here is also part of getting well. They think, 'I need to get well, I have to sit here, and I can share my experiences with someone else.' They talk, and ask each other how many times they have been coming. In this way they get relief from conversation, so people enjoy sitting here. That is why we want to make the waiting in an enjoyable space."*

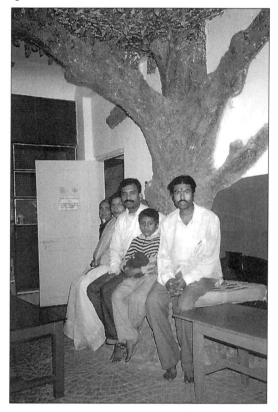

Waiting room

The doctor felt patients often waited so long to see him, that he wanted them to have a pleasant place, with tea facilities. Both the consulting room and the waiting room had an attached toilet. Patients often came huge distances to attend this surgery, sometimes up to 200 km. Patients wore their best clothes, good saris and finely decorated shawls. Together with their relatives they waited between four to six hours to see the psychiatrist.

While patients were waiting, a young man, Ariram, acting as receptionist and gatekeeper sang songs to them, some of which he had composed himself. He was a former patient who had been offered work as part of his rehabilitation. He took people's names, and kept them in order. There was also a therapist who had a side room to work in. He offered acupuncture in order to relieve mental distress. This was useful for migraine, anxiety, insomnia, withdrawal from alcohol or heroin, smoking, psychogenic impotence, alopecia, arthritic pains, and Parkinson's disease. He also offered psycho-drama therapy. The psychiatrist's intention was to integrate western medicine with eastern healing practices.

Consulting room. In the consulting room, one wall was made into a picture shrine of the spiritual practitioners of the Mother and Sri Aurobindo. One day, the arrival of a huge 4 foot high photograph of Sri Aurobindo in his advanced age, was ceremonially heralded by the continuous blowing of a conch shell. There were also pictures of the flower-laden *samadhi* (tomb) at Pondicherry and the Matri Mandir crystal ball at Auroville. There were fresh flowers everywhere: yellow and white chrysanthemums, and spikes of red gladioli. Over the desk there was another huge portrait of Sri Aurobindo as a young man. On other walls there were huge framed pictures of the Mother and Sri Aurobindo, embellished with garlands of scented flowers. In the consulting room there was a tape recorder, which constantly played gentle music, or organ music of the Mother. The doctor did no advertising: he said patients only came by the grace of the sage Sri Aurobindo and the Mother.

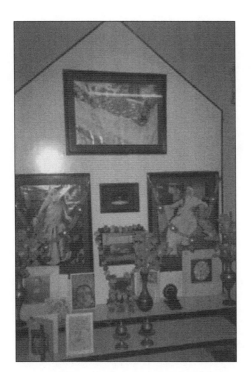

Shrine in the consulting room

The doctor practised within a western knowledge base, plus the addition of prayer and divine intervention of the Mother and Sri Aurobindo. The latter's relics (hair and nail clippings) were kept at the *Bhavan* in central Kolkata. The Mother allowed them to be sent out from Pondicherry on condition they received a full state honouring by the Indian government, which they did. They had been taken to Kolkata, Sri Aurobindo's birthplace, on a special journey because they had such a high vibration. They were then housed in a marble *samadhi*.

In the doctor's consulting room, Dr Basu sat behind a huge desk, and as well as seating for his patients, their relatives and neighbours, there were also stools or standing space for others. This included nine students of counselling and mental health, in their second year of a Master's degree. (They were from the social work department of Vidyasagar University, Salt Lake Campus, and helped by taking case studies and histories from patients in the waiting areas.)

When certain clients were ushered into his consulting room, the psychiatrist called in all nine students, as well as myself, plus his secretary who walked in and out, as did Ariram his receptionist. Consultation was more often a community activity, not just an individual process.

During the day pharmaceutical sales people came in, offering their ware from fine coloured books. They were smooth talking and humble, some very obsequious. Sometimes they offered the doctor fine incentives to buy their medicine, like train journeys, holidays, or other perks. However, the only thing he ever asked was that they gave a certain proportion of the drugs to him free, so he could offer them to his poor patients for nothing. In the consulting room, there was a large bag containing piles of the free drugs.

Locked Nursing Home. On Wednesday we visited another place in Kolkata where Dr Basu worked: the Sandipani Home. We took a taxi, driven by one of his former patients. During this first visit, SriRam, the astrologer also came to the nursing home with us, and added what he could 'see' clairvoyantly about the case histories. This place was a locked private nursing home, constructed on three floors with accommodation for nursing around fifteen men on the first floor, and ten women on the second. It had a pleasant tiled reception area, with a Hindu shrine facing the entrance. It cost relatives 200 rupees a day for patients to stay, and included the cost of the attendants and all meals.

The staff looked cheerful. Patients who came here were all under compulsory restraint. They had been violent, a danger to others in their communities, or had self-destructive behaviour. All those within had received a chemical pharmaceutical cosh in order to restrain them. The doctor kept them in the nursing home, away from their extended families, so they had the possibility of retrospection and looking inwards to consider their situation. I was told this kind of nursing home (where people could afford to send relatives) was being phased out.

The doctor told me in the past, 'schizophrenics' (his words) were kept in the prisons, where they had lived all their lives, with gardens and more space than other prisoners. Reformers moved them into locked lunatic asylums, built along a similar design, with wards off a central 'watchtower', but where they had less space, so it was not to their advantage. "*All of the old mental institutions in India were built in the pattern of jails. The jails had a central watchtower, with radial rooms. All these were from a time when there were no psychiatric medicines and people had to be confined. This tradition is now dying and we have to change. We are unable to have the infrastructure, for such institutions cannot be run on purely commercial grounds. We are in a terminal phase, and we need to be shifting to a central place for such institutions. Now we are planning places with plenty of gardens, where patients can be kept at low cost.*"

There are proposals for a centre of psychological health to be built at Auroville. The new project would be a residential healing centre for the treatment and investigation of psychological disorders based on Sri Aurobindo's philosophy on integral psychology, and on the principles of sacred architecture.

The psychiatrist checked over all the men in the Nursing home, and recorded their blood pressure. An older man there had been bereaved, and once his wife died, he couldn't cope with the isolation and turned to alcohol. His relatives had brought him in 35 days earlier. There was also another younger man, who spoke English, with a refined face, who had been addicted to 'brown sugar' (heroin). Three other young men all stood at the back of the room with their arms folded and their eyes staring. Two had been heroin addicts and had stolen from their families in order to buy drugs. One smaller youth, described as a schizophrenic, was violent and had been brought in chained with four padlocks, and had still managed to escape. He had no drug withdrawal symptoms, but was just extremely violent. After he treated the men, we left the nursing home and returned to the doctor's house.

When Dr Basu, myself and another colleague returned to the house I became very cold, frozen to the core. I thought I had food poisoning, laid on the bed and felt utterly miserable. It felt like I'd been hit by the chemical cosh of the nursing home men, and the violent energy that was being suppressed. Later I calmed down and my body heat returned. That night I had dreams that seemed to come from many thousands of years earlier. I had visions of many people entering a golden chamber, where all past lives and karmic deeds were burnt away by fire, watched by a host of non-incarnate beings. I woke up peacefully the following morning.

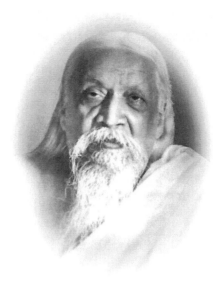

Sri Aurobindo

Journey to the Bangladesh Borders

Sunday clinics. The psychiatrist ran two clinics on a Sunday in a rural area inhabited mainly by Muslims, near the Bangladesh borders. We drove off there one Sunday in a small white van, on a family expedition, accompanied by the doctor's wife and his mother, and several baskets containing lots of food. Three hours later we reached the town of Basirat. We were going to travel on later to the village of Jhuruli, to meet a Muslim cleric who had been sending patients to Dr Basu's clinic for the last 10 years. We got out the car, and as we walked in the street, about to go up a flight of stairs to the clinic, I noticed a beautiful dove grey cat with soft fur, curled up sleeping immediately outside the entrance of the building. It seemed rather still. It looked perfectly calm, and at peace. The doctor's wife shouted at me *"Don't look at it, don't look at it..!"* It was perfectly dead.

The chamber was held in a small first floor hall, the far end of which was screened off with a plum coloured curtain. Behind this Dr Basu sat, with his assistants, and it was here that his patients went once they were called. In the waiting room there were half a dozen benches, with about 20 people: a relative or friend accompanied every patient. Some families brought in snacks, which they shared with others waiting. The consultation was quick, and in fact if these patients required a longer time to talk with him, he asked them to attend one of his clinics in Kolkata. Each patient had their blood pressure read, their prescription revised, and their condition updated. The doctor tried to see people quickly since he was aware that some had over 100 km to go in order to return home. He had a reputation for successful treatment, and patients knew he would offer treatments for no fees if they were poor. He and his wife were greatly respected by the patients.

In the waiting area I sat next to two men who had travelled from Bangladesh across the border with passports. One had been a heroin addict, a Muslim, who had been successfully treated so he brought his Hindu friend who was also an addict. They each had passports, but previously a prescription from the doctor himself served as a kind of passport to allow the state boundaries to be crossed. Furthermore, the doctor could adjust their length of stay, depending on how many weeks of treatment were needed.

Visit to holy man Haji Saheb

After the first clinic in Basirhat, we prepared to drive to the village of the Muslim cleric, Haji Saheb. We picked up two men to escort us there who had both been patients of Dr Basu. One was Mohammad, a painter of advertising boards, and the other was a mathematician who'd had a break down. They accompanied us for another hour's drive through the wetlands to the village. We travelled to the village of Jhuruli near the border with Bangladesh, about 20 km away, in the district of North 24 Pagonas in Bengal.

This village was in the waterways area, and was inhabited by shrimp and prawn farmers. There was water everywhere. The 'road' was a raised track between lakes, barely widely enough for the van's wheels: one slip and we would have toppled over the edge. I prayed to an unknown god while we drove. Raised mud walls defined different inhabitant's fish farming areas, and on the lake edges, thorny branches had been placed vertically in rows, to stop anyone using a net to trawl the waters and steal fish. Each of the wide water lakes had shelters for security watchmen.

These were small huts on stilts with low ridge roofs, built into the water, from where a farmer could watch over his stretch of lake throughout the night, and see off any pilferers and poachers. Some residential homes were themselves built on stilts over the water, with shallow tiled roofs.

When we arrived at the village of Jhuruli, our van was immediately surrounded by scores of people. The spiritual leader there, a Muslim cleric called Al Haji Saheb frequently sent people to Dr Basu for psychiatric care. However, the two men had never met. I was curious as to how he knew which patients to treat himself with spiritual and religious rituals and which to send to the psychiatrist. We were ushered into a side room in order to wait to speak to the cleric. We sat in this shaded room with most of the villagers looking through the doors and ventilation holes at us.

The spiritual leader or *molovi*, was working on a raised plinth, sheltered by an open walled ridged roof. In the centre of this space were two desks, with the Muslim cleric sitting on one side and two assistants on the other, each writing notes on small strips of white paper. Seated on benches around the tables and on the plinth, were the sick and suffering, and the disaffected, who were seeking healing or divination, quietly waiting their turn for an audience. The place had an atmosphere like a professional doctor's waiting room. The *molovi* was a man in his late 60's, with a long white beard. He had soft gentle eyes behind large glasses, and wore a blue chequered lunghi, and skullcap.

The elderly cleric stopped his surgery for a while in order to talk to us, and he agreed to be interviewed with Dr Basu on cassette, even though the younger clerics accompanying him clearly disapproved. His house was fronted by an open veranda, inside was the hall where we sat, and beyond was a huge open garden and courtyard with fruit trees. He had a wife, five boys and six girls, mostly grown up. Today was the first time the medical psychiatrist and the occultist therapist had ever met each other, even though they had seen each other's patients for some ten years.

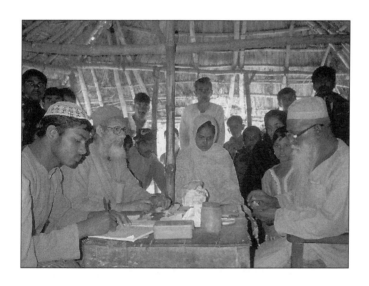

Consultation at cleric's clinic

Holy man's interpretation of Spirit possession. The Muslim cleric had been sending mental health patients to Dr Basu's clinic for years. He had a way of judging patients, to know which was a psychiatric case and which was curable by Islamic rituals. Once he had done the appropriate rituals, he sent the person on to Dr Basu for treatment. He treated cases of possession and other illnesses caused by spirit, but he sent psychiatric cases to the clinic. People came to him across great distances to resolve their health and social problems. He had sent a number of people to the psychiatrist, those he said he could not help with religious or occult means.

I asked the Molovi how he distinguished between those people coming to him who needed religious or spiritual treatment, and those who needed psychiatric treatment. I asked him to define how he distinguished between the symptoms of mental illness and spirit possession. I didn't speak his language, so Dr Basu translated his words: *"He differentiates between what he feels is organic mental illness and possession states. If it is a case of spirit possession he takes steps here. Those he thinks are pure mental patients he sends to my clinic. There are certain symptoms, which he describes. He discriminates on the basis of symptoms. If it is a spirit possession state, he can see partly a sign in the head, partly a sign in the eyes, and partly a sign in the hands."*

If he did encounter a person with a possession state, he treated them by giving specific charms or amulets (*taviiz*), which could be worn around the arm, neck or waist. *"He sees which one is suited for whom, for he also has to differentiate. It is not the same for everyone. It depends on the individual cases. It depends on different diseases and the intensity of the diseases, that the charms are given."*

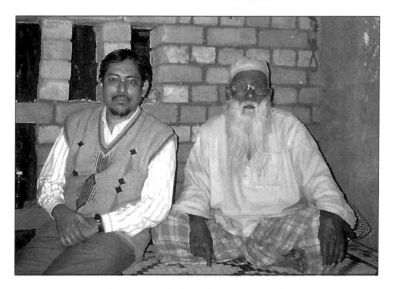

Dr Basu and the molovi Haji Saheb

Causes of possession. I wanted to know what the cause was of a possession state, and I wondered how the *Molovi* had become skilled at defining them. Dr Basu translated his words "*There are beings of another world, who have different types of bodies, subtle bodies. They move in subtle ether. They move in ethereal space. Sometimes they come and influence people. They have a bad influence on human beings, and that causes illness. These beings are of a different world, of a different dimension, which we usually cannot visualise. But they are there, though he says people might not believe it, that these beings are there, and it is their bad influence that can cause these illnesses. An act of illness may be manifested in the sort of attacks we see that give fits and fever, where the eyeballs roll up... This is a serious type.*"

The Molovi explained it was possible to visualise these subtle beings through practise, and they were not solid. They were more like an impression, or a silhouette. He gained his training through another teacher, and he developed the skills himself through his own practice and experience. I was still unclear how he could diagnose which patients were psychiatric, and I wondered what the symptoms were. "*He differentiates the spirit possession ones from the signs of their hands, their eyes, and their language. And when he doesn't get those signs, then he sends those people to our clinic."*

The Molovi noticed people responded well to Dr Basu's psychiatric treatments, and had continued to send patients there for the last ten years. For example in the 1990's, he had sent a young man to the psychiatrist. This was Mohammed, a cheerful person I had met earlier. He was brought to the cleric in an aggressive violent state. He was carried in by his village men folk, but he couldn't remember anything about it. The Molovi said: *"immediately I recognised it, by seeing those symptoms, like self-muttering. (He is talking about all the schizophrenic symptoms here: gesturing, posturing, the way they moved their eyes.) He immediately said these are not possession states and require real treatment by drugs."* Dr Basu continued: *"Actually he is doing a great service by differentiating them. So he just sends me those specific cases which are relevant."*

I wondered how this kind of work related to the teachings in the Koran. Dr Basu translated: *"there are specific norms about living in the Koran, like the way you should eat, the way you should perform your daily ablutions. If you deviate from the norms, if you go and do your daily things in a way you should not, then occult forces might influence you. The Koran gives a base, of seed ideas, from which he constructs his sadana (spiritual pursuits) and aradana (medical practice and rituals, as part of one's religious or spiritual work). He takes up the seed ideas from the Koran, he takes up the spirituality from the Koran, and he develops it into his own sadana. He is saying it is not only reading but he has to develop practice as well"* (sadana is the practice of cultivating spirituality).

The Molovi asked me whether we recognised and acknowledged cases of spirit possession in England. I explained in the west, psychiatry had defined a series of symptoms, and apart from organic brain malfunction, it did not appear to be able to define causation in that way. When some psychiatrists retired in their late 60's and 70's, some seemed to realise they didn't always know causes of mental illness (Sanderson[28], Powell[29]) and came to spiritual conclusions. I told him there were very few practitioners who recognised or accepted a diagnosis of spirit possession, although I was aware certain psychiatrists were exploring this aspect (Bhugra[30], Bhui[31], Dein[32]).

The Molovi explained "*in spirit possession, it is a cause of psychiatric symptoms, and psychiatrists only treat the symptoms. In such cases the symptoms will be resolved, but the possession will remain and might affect the person in some other way.*" I had heard of practitioners from other countries who had said similar things (for example the shaman Malidome Some[33], and the psychiatrist Kharitidi[34]). In the west, there seemed to be two streams of thought regarding health: biological medicine and spiritual strategies which used a subtle approach, of people who could see like shamans and psychics, but kept silent. I felt there had been very little bridging between them.

I had wanted to work in India, because the bridge between different professionals who dealt in health already appeared to be present in some cases. I was glad to see the two of them in person, working together even though they had never met before. Dr Basu said "*the day is coming in future where the bridging will happen. Sri Aurobindo has said that is the next stage, the age of subjectivity, when science and mysticism will come closer.*" I asked the Molovi whether he had any inhibitions about taking help from scientific research, as he himself was a mystic. He replied "*Let sadana (spiritual pursuit) and gavesana (scientific research) exist together. What is the harm in that?*"

I had come to this village across many waterways, seeing architecture I'd never seen before, land and water new to me. After so many hours of driving when we arrived here, we saw the Molovi's patients sitting quietly under the shade. It had the atmosphere of a doctor's surgery. It was very calm, very quiet, and very professional. Dr Basu said of the Molovi "*he has such a nice vibration and a clear aura: people get energised by him*".

I was pleased to see the two men together, one who represented the medical aspect of psychiatry, and the other who represented the subtle aspect of psychiatry, both sitting together in one room. It felt very good.

Upon leaving, the Molovi gave us blessings to keep ourselves in good health. "*He has blessed us so that the Almighty's Light is upon us, and that we should be better off. And the way we have been working we should continue to work in cooperation.*"

Later in the day, after we left the Molovi, thanking him for his hospitality, we drove on again. The doctor held a second chamber later that same day at Bera Champa. He was concerned that if this chamber ran late, his patients had to travel across rivers and tiger infested forest, taking several hundred kilometres to reach home. He checked on patients quickly and updated their programme. Once the clinics were over, we drove back to Kolkata, arriving in the early hours.

Watching from the Kolkata balcony

The following morning before breakfast, I sat on the second-floor balcony for a while, trying to get warm in the cool morning sun. Opposite there was a sign for an art gallery, open for business. The sign barely hung on the wall. In the street below, the egg merchant arrived with a cart full of eggs in cardboard boxes. He rang a bell at street level. From the fifth floor balcony, one woman leaned out and lowered down an orange bucket on a very long rope. The salesman filled it with the required number of eggs, and then she drew the bucket, hauling up her merchandise, and walked back in closing the shutters.

On the road, a man walked up and down strumming a single string: announcing that he made pillows and carded cotton for mattresses. In another apartment further down the road, two women with shiny black hair, drew a bucket of fresh spinach leaves up to their balcony using a long rope, which they bought from a salesman in the street five stories below.

In the afternoon, I sat outside on the balcony, and wrote up my notes. I noticed some homes had an iron grille half way around the balcony, whereas in other places the grille was full height, like a security cage around their home. People hung their washing out on it, blowing in the wind, several storeys above the street. On the balcony opposite, a pair of eyes peeped out from amongst the suspended washing. They met my eyes. I didn't know whether to smile in acknowledgement or not. I didn't know whether the peering eyes wanted to be seen.

I went up to the roof. From there, it was possible to see the sunset, just after 5.00 pm, with a beautiful view of palm trees, water ponds and birds like kingfishers, green parrots, and many sparrows and crows. The sun went down quickly in a misty sky, a gentle glowing red orb across this cityscape of apartment blocks.

That evening after dark, I went with the doctor's wife into town to a fish market, travelling in a cycle rickshaw through the dusty streets. The covered market was lit by naked light bulbs, and some small fish were still flapping, alive in low water. By 9.30 pm most of the fish-mongers were scrubbing up. While we were waiting for our fish to be scaled and sliced into cutlets, I saw a man in the row behind plucking a freshly slaughtered bird. Behind him was a cage of live chickens. He reached into it, took out a bird, weighed it, and it squawked until he cut its throat. Then silence. It only took a few seconds. Then he skinned it completely, washed his hands in a bucket, and wiped them on a rag, all in a couple of minutes. We took the fish and caught an auto-rickshaw home and had a very late supper.

I went to bed mulling over the last few intense days. I'd started out on a 36 hour train journey from Chennai to Kolkata. I'd visited Dr Basu's psychiatric clinics both in Kolkata, and on the Bangladesh borders. Also I'd seen the locked nursing home, which was the equivalent of 'private' paying health care, for those whose families could afford it. I found there was a peaceful informal atmosphere in waiting areas for patients and their families, sustained by both the psychiatrist and also by the Muslim cleric we visited. I was surprised the two men had never met before our visit, as they had been sharing clients for ten years.

Life in Kolkata felt raw and crowded, an assault on my senses. I was extremely grateful that I was staying in the family home. In the following days, Dr Basu said he would allow me to interview some of his patients, so that I could understand their perspectives on health.

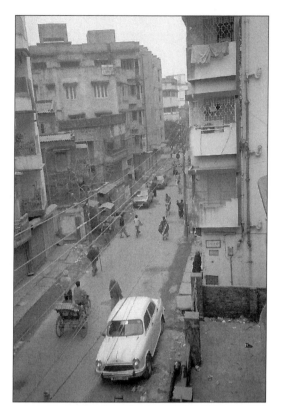

Bangur Avenue balcony

Chapter Three

INTERVIEWS WITH PATIENTS

Introduction

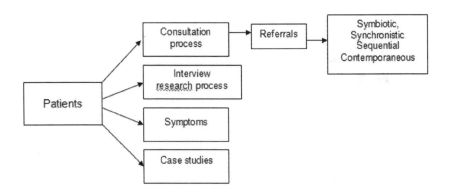

I interviewed patients and observed the consultation process, noting referrals that took place between practitioners. Some patient referrals were symbiotic occurring by the agency of two mutually understanding practitioners, or the taking of treatments that worked well together. Other referrals were synchronistic and contemporaneous, that is consultations occurred within the same time period. Then there were referrals that took place sequentially, one after the other.

On some days I sat in the psychiatrist's consulting room in Kolkata for several hours at a time, observing Dr Basu's practice alongside the nine social work students. He would work for hours on end, without resting, and during this time, he allocated certain patients for me to talk to. The first time I went to Kolkata, he allocated more male than female patients, and when I commented on this, he rectified the balance during a later visit.

One thing was overwhelmingly clear: an individual consultation involved the client, his or her spouse, parents or grandparents, the nine students, myself, a receptionist and secretary who came in during the consultation. An individual consultation did not mean the one to one private encounter we see in the west. There could be up to 18 people in the room at the same time. This was quite unlike the one to one individual consultations in the west.

The taking of case histories by the clinical assistants in the waiting room, was in itself considered a therapeutic act, as was the hearing and acknowledging of that case history, repeated in front of the psychiatrist. The students were usually responsible for doing this and reporting back. As mentioned earlier, the process of waiting was also considered to be therapeutic, and the waiting areas were made as pleasant as possible. There was no appointment system, apart from the given day, and patients were seen in the order in which they arrived. Dr Basu believed discussions among patients in the waiting area were like co-counselling and helped to relieve the stress of the carers and add to the healing experience. The waiting area was designed to promote a sense of calmness in patients and their carers: it was intended to be a healing space.

Interviews

Patients selected for interview were chosen by the psychiatrist, and depended on the days I visited his clinic, and who was present at the time. I spoke no Bengali, so different people translated discussions, and sometimes filtering of content occurred. Sometimes I conducted the interviews in the doctor's house, and sometimes in rooms within his clinics. These locations could have influenced or biased the kinds of answers I received, but there was no other option. I interviewed a total of 25 patients, 13 women and 12 men, each of whom was allocated by the psychiatrist, depending on the day I was present and who he had in the clinic.

I recorded which patients were single, married, or divorced, since subsequently I would explore the triggers for mental ill health according to these categories. Sampling was purposive: the main aim at the time was to provide opportunities for me to interview as many people as possible before I was called back urgently to the UK, due to the clairvoyantly seen, prophesied, and assumed imminent death of my mother.

In some cases I would speak directly with the patients if they knew English. However, if I could not speak to patients directly (I had no Bengali), then the doctor asked one of his social workers to translate, or his wife, or Ariram, one of his rehabilitated patients. Some patients understood English even though they preferred to be interviewed in their own language.

Obviously my not speaking Bengali risked problems of interpretation, or the filtering of socially acceptable responses to my questions. In one case with Ariram, while interviewing a couple (no.25), I was aware the answers were being edited. In fact they were edited to such a huge extent, and the responses so garbled, that I called a halt to the interview. Once the couple in question had left the room, Ariram was more explicit and told me their story was a shocking one about female infidelity within marriage.

There were other problems: on another occasion, a patient let out a flow of rapid Bengali in response to my question, and as soon as the translator started explaining in English, she swiftly continued in Bengali. It was very difficult to catch her story. Other patients seemed relieved to talk to me, as if unburdening themselves of their anguish. One woman commented: "*I feel so much glad talking to you. After a long time I didn't talk so much with anyone.*" Perhaps she hadn't received enough counselling for her own requirements.

Consultation

Dr Basu's psychiatric clinics were private: fee paying for those who could afford it, and free to those who could not (about a third of patients were charity cases). The doctor said his cured patients were his best advertisement. Patients sometimes travelled hundreds of miles to attend his clinics. However, by the time they came to see him, they had often tried a number of other practitioners including physicians, priests, and traditional healers. General physicians, other psychiatrists, astrologers, and religious leaders often referred patients to him. The W.H.O. (World Health Organisation) wanted physicians to co-operate with traditional healers, so they could be in contact with all kinds of people.

Patients tended to consult medical specialists sequentially, trying out different ones and assessing the results. However, sometimes they saw religious or traditional healers contemporaneously, that is, they felt their treatments would work in a complementary fashion, alongside bio-medicine. Their responses were pragmatic: they saw no point in taking pharmacological products if they didn't modify their social relationships, or built environment at the same time; or if they didn't appease spiritual influences of the planets or local deities, effects of karma, or trans-generational influences, with appropriate rituals.

Practitioners consulted by mental health patients
- Priests
- Psychiatrists
- Psychologists
- Medical herbalists
- Homoeopaths
- Traditional healers (oja)
- Traditional teacher (guru)
- Astrologers
- Vastusilpi (architectural specialist)

Many patients felt the treatments were symbiotic and worked well in combination. They consulted astrologers in order to determine any steps they should take to appease the planetary systems, and architectural specialists for advice on modifying their homes or compounds to ameliorate their mental health. Usually they consulted with a physician or a psychiatrist sequentially, or would be referred onwards. There were also referrals between different types of practitioner. There were examples of physicians and traditional healers referring clients to psychiatrists, and psychiatrists referring patients to their medical colleagues, or to indigenous healers. Going for a consultation was itself considered as part of the treatment strategy. Often patients came in their best clothes for their appointment. For example one woman (no.22), had come to the clinic in a red sari, wore lots of jewellery and had three amulets on her arm *(taviz)*. She was from a Hindu family, but had visited a Muslim traditional healer as well as the psychiatrist.

Thus patients used a multiplicity of consultation strategies. They either consulted different practitioners singly, sequentially or contemporaneously. They felt each treatment influenced different aspects of their ill health or symptoms, and some could be used contemporaneously. If their condition also required a religious or ritual input, patients would undertake these alongside consuming pharmacological products. They would also consult astrologers or palm readers to throw light on what was happening to them. During my visit to South India, I discovered many people visited the town of Vaitheeswarakoil, to consult with the Palm Leaf Oracle libraries (see chapters 5, 6, and 7 on Treatment Strategies). This helped them to contextualise their illness event, and the oracles suggested rituals to perform in the surrounding shrines or temples. There were several examples, of patients consulting with traditional healers or gurus in temples, and religious leaders of various faiths, their own and others.

Dr Basu (who received patient referrals from shamans and traditional healers) gave one example, of a female patient in a highly psychotic state. An occultist had told him she was wearing hidden amulets that affected her behaviour, and they needed to be removed. This was something he would not have otherwise known. For example, when one woman's symptoms first started after marriage, her father took her to see an occultist, a traditional healer or '*oja*'. He performed some rituals, said mantras, blew air and sprays of water onto her, and prepared amulets. "*Water was given to her which was charmed with mantras: it was blown over her.*" After that her father was told that hers was no longer a case, which could be dealt with by an occultist, she had to come under the domain of a psychiatrist. "*The oja said 'whatever I have had to do, I have done, now it comes under the domain of psychiatry. You had better consult a specialist.'*

| | | | | CHART 3.1 | | |
| | | | | THE PATIENTS | | |
No.	Initial		Age	Accompanied by...	Religion (& caste)	Occupation
1	SB	M	37	not known	Hindu (Brahmin)	rehabilitation working at doctor's clinic
2	Ar	M	33	not known	Hindu kayestu)	rehabilitation working at doctor's clinic
3	MSAM	M	33	10-12 villagers (10 years ago)	Muslim	sign-writer
4	AS	M	24	In Nursing Home	Hindu (kayestu)	
5	PD	F	26	Husband	Hindu (vaiysha)	
6	M	M	40's	Alone	Hindu (vaiysha)	Singer: devotional songs
7	SC	M	44	Alone	Hindu (Brahmin)	librarian
8	NB	M	28	not known	Hindu (kayestu)	Social work student
9	KM	F	30	Mother	Hindu	
10	MS	M	16	In Nursing home	Hindu	
11	HS	M	40's	not known	Hindu (shedule)	Lawyer in his village
12	AB	M	20's	not known	Hindu	
13	MH	F	42	Husband	Hindu	
14	MS	F	24	Mother	Hindu	
15	CB	F	22	Parents, grandparents	Hindu (brahmin)	Engineering student
16	MRS	F	32	Husband	Hindu (Brahmin)	Government job
17	RS	F	29	Parents	Hindu (shedule)	
18	SR	F	17	Mother	Hindu (kayestu)	
19	MS	F	23	Mother & sister	Hindu (kayestu)	
20	KP	M	29	Mother, sister's husband	Hindu (Mahishya)	
21	RP	M	25	Brothers	Hindu (vaisha)	
22	NS	F	35	Husband	Hindu (kayestu)	
23	SR	F	33	Husband	Hindu (kayestu)	
24	JS	F	34		Hindu (kayestu)	
25	RN	F	30	Husband	Hindu (kayestu)	

Patients

Patients I interviewed ranged from 16 to 44 years old, with 13 women seen and 12 men. Of the six married women, each one was accompanied to the clinic by their husband. Dr Basu suggested for a number of women, their husband's sincerity in following the treatment procedure and follow-up visit to the clinic was a major factor in their mental stability. He felt some husbands were more concerned about their wife's well-being than the woman herself. Dr Basu observed "*women and girls with psychiatric problems can be in a very difficult situation, since they carry the honour and shame for their family.*" This shame did not extend to a man with psychiatric problems. The chart 3.1 illustrates the gender, age and religion of patients, together with their occupation.

Single women were accompanied by their mothers and sisters, and in one case by both sets of grandparents as well. Only one Muslim patient was interviewed from the Basirhat clinic, and the majority rest were Hindu, with many belonging to the Brahmin (priestly) and Kayestu (warrior) caste. Many were from the educated, upper and middle class levels of society. Where known, patients' occupations are given. Two of Dr Basu's former patients were working in his clinics as part of their rehabilitation programme, and others did this voluntarily for the Basirhat clinics, as part of their grateful service to the psychiatrist. Of those patients mentioned below, six had been under compulsory restraint in the Nursing home, only one was a woman.

Symptoms

The patients I interviewed mentioned a series of symptoms that included emotional and physiological conditions, impairment of faculties, and 'abnormal' behaviour. The emotions included anger, jealousy, feeling depressed, having no joy in life, being morose, and feeling despair from loss of trust in close relatives. The somatic indicators were headaches, tiredness, tension, fainting, fever, chest pains, problems breathing, insomnia, not being able to eat or sleep, experiencing body shaking and trembling. Patients experienced some impairment to their 'normal' human faculties and these included: memory loss, hearing sounds, having hallucinations, and sudden bouts of unconsciousness.

CHART 3.2
RANGE OF SYMPTOMS

ACCORDING TO PATIENTS INTERVIEWED

- Anger, jealousy, depression, no joy in life, morose
- Tiredness, fainting, chest pains, problems breathing, insomnia, not eating or sleeping, headaches, body shaking, fever, tension
- Memory loss, hearing sounds, having hallucinations, sudden bouts of unconsciousness, can't recognise own belongings, unable to work, lack of concentration
- Screaming and throwing things, crying, violence towards parents, violence towards sibling
- Self-harm, attempted suicide (jumping into a well, walking on railways tracks, hanging),

PLUS... ACCORDING TO PRACTITIONERS

(for specific diagnoses see below)

- Obsessive behaviour, repeated rituals, perversions, sexual aberrations, rebelliousness, violence, psychotic, paranoid, delusional, grandiosity, confusion, withdrawal from social interaction, meaningless talk

---

Some patients were unable to recognise their own belongings, or unable to work, lacking in concentration. Others had 'abnormal behaviour' which manifested in the following ways: screaming and throwing things, crying, exhibiting violence towards their parents or siblings. A number had tried to self-harm, or had attempted suicide (by jumping into a well, walking on railways tracks at night, or attempted hanging). Practitioners added the following: behaviour that was obsessive, psychotic, violent, paranoid, delusional, grandiose, or confusional. According to Dr Basu, there were also those who withdrew from all social interaction, muttered meaningless speech, repeated mundane or religious rituals, had perversions or sexual aberrations, or were rebellious.

Meeting Patients

I was interested to hear about peoples beliefs on the triggers for mental distress, and the strategies that doctor and patients used to achieve health. The first few patients mentioned here attended open clinics, but later interviews were with patients in the locked nursing home. The last patient mentioned was referred from the Muslim Cleric. I have given selected descriptions of only a few patients below.

The Psychotic Psychic. The first patient I was invited to interview was SriRam, the clairvoyant astrologer mentioned at the beginning of this chapter, who gave me the unsolicited reading. The interview was held in the sitting room of Dr Basu's home, in front of all his guests. I found this was one of the most difficult interviews, since it was interspersed with unsolicited prophesies about myself and members of my family that were quite shocking. By the end of it I felt as if my life had been stripped bare, and I even had to be careful what thoughts passed through my mind. When he spoke everyone in the room could hear what he said, whether it was the number of conceptions my mother had, whether or not I should take a lover, and whether or not I had occult (hidden) abilities. I received answers to questions I had not asked, and would not have asked.

Sri Ram spoke only Bengali, and I spoke to him with Dr Basu translating my questions and his answers. He used to work in a shoe shop and began having clairvoyant experiences in 1997 when he saw people's faces he realised he could tell their future. Some experiences were beneficial and others were negative. Although he called himself an astrologer (a catch-all term for clairvoyant / psychic), he had no idea how astrology worked. When he visited the palm leaf oracles, they confirmed that whatever he said was the truth. He had been one of Dr Basu's patients for manic depressive psychosis, and was still on a maintenance dose of lithium.

He discovered his gift for prophesying the future in 1997 and he helped couples achieve fertility, and lawyers win their court cases. Each day about 100-150 people would come to him. After the sudden death of both his parents, he felt his gift to others was like a curse on himself, so he went to a *tantric* priest to get initiation. The *tantric* priest he saw at Tirol temple in West Bengal had undertaken rituals involving the skull of a dead person at a burial ground, which was used particularly for occult purposes.

SriRam was given a substance by mouth, which he ingested and he felt it was this that subsequently caused a mental break down. The substance was a paste made of herbs, brain of a dead owl, and ashes of a burnt corpse, which was drunk with tea. This made him mentally ill and he came to the psychiatrist's attention. He had two manic attacks and one attack of mild depression, and was diagnosed as a case of manic depressive psychosis. He had attacks of manic phases whenever he strained himself too much in astrological work, and made too many correct predictions. He was maintained on Valproate, a mood stabiliser and had been advised restraint in his astrological work.

This kind of swinging alternation between a gifted state and a psychiatric state is common in the literature[35] and there are web blogs devoted to the continuum of psychosis and spirituality[36], [37]. SriRam attended the clinic and was used by the psychiatrist for his gift of prophesy, to provide additional information on other patients' condition, or to conduct prayer rituals on their behalf. Sri Ram felt very comfortable in Dr Basu's company and had come to appreciate Sri Aurobindo and the Mother's energy through him. Due to his gifts of clairvoyance he assisted in the surgery with spiritual advice in some cases.

Dr Basu and his wife introduced me to another patient M.Ranjan, who was resident at the same temple mentioned by SriRam. This was at Tirol in Tarapith, a temple that was one of the foremost places for occultism in India. It was a place where initiates meditated on corpses in the funeral ground. This place was dedicated to the goddess Kali, with a big funeral ground where occult rituals took place. (In India the word occult does not have the same pejorative meaning as in the west. It means 'that which is hidden', in the same way clairvoyants can see what is hidden beyond the five senses. Hidden aspects or practices might be good or bad.)

After that shocking experience of being prophesied at by SriRam, I wondered exactly what these clairvoyants were seeing around me. Were they seeing some potential future event, which may not manifest? Were they seeing events from my own personal existence or history, or were they tuning into events of some other entity, which was projecting something, to make me feel uneasy. One thing was very clear: there were absolutely no protocols for the safe offering of clairvoyant information. I felt very vulnerable.

The Dutiful Daughter. The following morning, I was invited to meet a young woman in her 30's, who had tried to hang herself the day before. I was taken into a side room in the chamber to interview her. Kalpina came in with her mother, a gentle smiling woman, and removed her scarf to show me the burn marks on her neck from the attempted hanging. Dr Basu's wife translated for us, from Bengali to English. She said Kalpina became anxious after she quarrelled with her neighbours (the family lived in a rented house with other tenants). She helped her mother in domestic work, and was the oldest child with a younger brother and sister. She had never married and first came to see the psychiatrist in her teens. At that time her hands trembled, she spoke very fast, and couldn't do her studies in school. She had repeatedly threatened and attempted suicide. Her mother had taken her to a guru in a temple for healing rituals. This helped but had not lasted. Her mother explained: "*where we are living, it is a rented house, people are very poor. There are slums. People are not satisfied, but they do not commit suicide.*" She continued: "*when she was young, she had seen someone committing suicide by hanging. Seeing this, it really affected her happiness on the mental plane. It affected her a bit, when she was small.*"

It was difficult for me to compute, the smiling girl in front of me, with one who had tried to hang herself the day before, together with her gently spoken apparently caring mother. Later it transpired there had been two unnatural deaths in the family. Although the triggers had been quarrels with neighbours, the seer SriRam suggested there may have been other influences. For example it might have been a disembodied being had jumped onto her, from a person who committed suicide nearby. In this way the pattern of someone who had killed themselves, could have become imprinted on her. If that first pattern could be removed, then perhaps she wouldn't attempt suicide anymore. He suggested she see an occultist, who could sense the original, which had occurred when she was small, and would remove the pattern itself. When the psychiatrist asked another astrologer to look at Kalpina energetically he confirmed she had an imprint from a deceased entity.

Dr Basu commented on her case saying: "*She has cycles of depression alternating with cycles where manic and paranoid symptoms coexist intensely. She has attempted suicide more than once. In between attacks, she is OK on a very low dose of maintenance medication (valpraote and trifluoperazine). In the interludes she is a loving, dutiful girl, and nobody would guess that she has psychiatric problems. She saw a suicide in childhood, and like her I have seen some other women who had seen suicide in childhood and later on these women had depressive spells."* He felt these childhood memories left impressions on his patients, and he believed that such cases would benefit from occult help in addition to western psychiatric treatment. He mentioned he wanted to develop trials for these kinds of cases, where psychiatric interventions would be used together with occult remedies recommended by experts. Additional rituals included praying, burning camphor, and the use of special stones charged with power from temples.

The Naxalite. There was another former patient who worked at the surgeries as part of his rehabilitation. Sometimes he translated when I interviewed other patients. Ariram was a softly spoken, slightly-built, refined looking, young man of 33. He had gentle features and was well educated, speaking impeccable English. He helped out in the surgery, registering the names of the patients, regulating the crowds, calling them into the consultation chamber, and singing to them in the waiting room to calm them. He sang Bengali songs in the psychiatrist's chamber in Kolkata, and Muslim songs about Mecca in the Basirhat clinic. He worked up to 10 hours a day, and his creative bent was used to offer music therapy and psychodrama sessions. He wrote poetry, composed songs, took good photographs and made documentary films. *"In the chamber, I register the names of patients, and the order they arrive in. They are seen first come, first served. There are no appointments only the date is given. Patients may wait up to four hours to see the doctor. Sometimes I assist the doctor to help patients talk, to get them out of the inhibitions. The doctor does the treatment."*

Dr Basu said Ariram had borderline personality disorder with a history of multiple substance abuse and deviancy, and streaks of schizoid thoughts. He rebelled against societal norms, and had an adjustment disorder with his family. *"His diagnosis does not fit into classical ICD10 and DSM IV grooves, and we have found that a holistic approach was more suited to work with him. He takes lithium, carbamazapine and clozapine in low doses, a combination which we found is suited as his maintenance medication. He remains well if he is on a very low dose of mood stabilisers. He takes a low dose of respiridol. If he doesn't take the medicine, his thinking patterns change, and he goes back to drugs, opiates, and cannabis. He has enormous personality problems. Has he told you about his stint with polyandry? To do that in today's world, you can understand the kind of mind he has. He has weird sexual aberrations."*

Ariram was from a Hindu *rajiru* (royal) background, but rejected his parent's caste philosophy and background when he was 15 years old. One of his classmates was a leftist with the CPIM (Communist Party of India Marxist). He became acquainted with Marxism and started going around with Naxalites. These were from a small place in the north of Bengal, where the nationalised government had fired upon a group of poor farmers who had died. Ariram was interested in politics and got into trouble at school: they were going to suspend him, but didn't and he passed his exams with good results. Then he met someone who introduced him to brown sugar (heroin) and polyandry. *"Polyandry?"* I asked. *"It is spelt..."* *"I know how it is spelt"* I replied *"but what does it mean?"* *"It means having sexual experiences with the same opposite sex, by many people, together, one by one, somehow."*

He came to Dr Basu's attention during the mid 1990's, and was kept in the nursing home for one year. *"When he went in he weighed 29 kgs. and he was taking 16-20 spasmoproximal tablets a day, a painkiller, which contains synthetic opiates."* Ariram said *"at that time I was totally broken in body and mind. I got broken after my divorce with my wife. I started drinking. In those days I used to lie in the road drunk. I used hallucinogens in the beginning, LSD. I had dreams and hallucinations, for I wanted to get away from the war and the tensions. I never had a bad trip. It was always beneficial. After that, I started taking heroin and other things, tranquillisers, and I used to drink. I took all kinds of mixtures of drugs and alcohol. After that, when I was broken, I just used to take alcohol and lie in the streets. My parents forced me to go to the doctor's."*

Ariram thought Dr Basu was a very unusual psychiatrist, and felt he had a spiritual aura around himself and in the clinic where they worked. *"I never thought a psychiatrist's chamber was a place where I could feel comfortable but when I met the doctor I got some other vibrations. That was the place I wanted to be. I got this vibration without using drugs, in Dr Basu's company with his fine gestures. Somehow I found a place and a vibration, which was the vibration of a metaphysical world. Then I stopped taking drugs, illegal drugs, but I used psychiatric drugs. What the drugs had done, I could do by myself. What the drugs could not do, I got from Dr Basu: a vibration that helped me have different visions which people will usually have when they take hallucinogens or grass....I first got the vibration in his company that I used to get in my old drug abusing days. That made him very unusual for me."*

Once the tape stopped he told me about the three times he'd been in a nursing home, about his drug addiction, alcohol abuse, and sleeping in the street. He was admitted to the Nursing home three times: at ages 17, 28, and 32. (Note: people often opened up more once the tape was turned off.) When the interview ended he sang one of his songs. He said it was a song about peace. *"If you take a hand grenade from people's hand, and in its place put a mandolin, and let the children rest on their mother's laps, and have sweet dreams, and the world is one country. Everyone should feel the love of songs and the love of flowers."*

Ill-treated daughter-in-law. On Tuesday I saw another female patient called Nalima, who said she had been to various gurus and traditional healers, unknown to her husband, who was surprised to hear about such things in the interview. She was suffering from depression, memory loss, and obsessive behaviour, triggered by poor treatment from her in-laws. She had been coming to see Dr Basu for the last two years, and his treatments had helped her. She had visited religious practitioners outside psychiatry including going to both a Hindu and a Muslim traditional healer (*oja*). They gave her amulets (*taviz*) to wear on her upper arm and neck. An aunt from her natal family first took her, and they were told that her in-laws had done 'something bad' to her.

The film star. The second boy I spoke to was sixteen years old, paranoid and delusional. He was brought down to talk to me. However, he was in such a stupor, that it didn't feel appropriate for me to ask about using the cassette to record the interview. He spoke directly with me in good English, said he hated being there, and wanted to go back to his mother and father. He had only been there one week, said he cried all night, and felt he was in a jail, imprisoned. When asked, he told me both his names: his own and that of a film star. I kept asking why he was there, and he repeatedly said he didn't know, but after a while said he had beaten up his mother. His parents could not control him and the doctor said the nursing home gave him a chance of introspection and reflection.

When he spoke it was in a quiet child's voice. The drugs held him in a stupor-like state, unmoving. He was Hindu, his parents were traders, and he had arrived in an acute psychotic state. His family were from a schedule caste (untouchables) and he had given himself a Bombay film star's name. He had given himself a different identity, with a different name and language. He spoke only Hindi though his native language was Bengali. He had disconnected from his family, and was very violent. He was aggressive towards his parents, refused to eat, suspicious and totally lost in a fantasy world of film stars. He hated to be identified with his father's under-garment business.

He was attached to his maternal uncle, a rich businessman who himself suffered from grandiose ideas (he had a manic episode once, and was diagnosed as having bipolar disorder). From childhood, the boy detested his father's social position, an attitude that increased by his association with his maternal uncle, and led to the current break down. The psychiatrist commented: "*he speaks fluent English, better than many, and in terms of knowledge and body language, seems almost a misfit in his social station. When a boy is such a misfit in his social class, and in addition learns to detest his parents, he may suffer a severe identity crisis that may lead to a psychotic break down. Sometimes in such cases, perhaps past life therapies would have a role in unravelling aspects of his background, which we little understand today.*" This was the fist time I had heard mention about past lives being an influence on present distress. I didn't ask what kind of therapies were available to address the condition.

The very nice boy. I was invited to talk to a number of inmates in the locked nursing home. I spoke to one chubby young man of 24, who came from a wealthy family and had lived off his father's money. He was compulsorily detained, with his family's blessings. When I met him, he was shaking uncontrollably from the drugs, his lips trembling, with his arms hanging limply on his lap. After his father's death, he experienced intense conflict and developed a paranoid disorder, and a disorder of impulse control. "*The boy has turned to spirituality but continues to harbour aggressive thoughts against his mother. In a fit of paranoia, he went to illegally purchase a gun without a licence. We felt he would kill his mother in a spell of delusion, so we had him admitted to this* *nursing home. Because he had turned towards spirituality, much of our counselling was directed to help this grow."* This young man was very aggressive towards his mother. He used money to go across state borders, buy a gun, and had then threatened his mother. He bought himself an apartment in Pondicherry so he could be near the Sri Aurobindo ashram.

The psychiatrist told us *"He is a very nice boy at heart, very spiritual. He has a combination of spirituality and psychosis, side by side"*. I interviewed him in English directly, in front of everyone. I had to keep asking questions, since he answered each one with just a phrase, or sentence. He never continued to talk. When the doctor questioned him about his drinking habits, and his decision to buy a gun, he started shaking uncontrollably again. When he went to write his name, his hand shook so much from heavy medication he couldn't write his own name. He spent 3 months 21 days inside. Dr Basu released him the day after the interview, since he felt he had shown remorse and awareness.

3.3
INTERVIEW WITH THE VERY NICE BOY

What are you doing here in Kolkata?

For this business I am here, otherwise I should have been in Pondicherry ashram.

What is this place, where we are now?

It is not a very good place.

Why?

Lots of drug addicts come here, and lots of anti social people.

And here, in this building, this room looks pleasant. What is this place?

Only these two rooms are kept so nicely for the doctors, but upstairs is not good, for the patients. It is not good for the patients to be here. It is not at all good for the patients.

Why?

It is not at all suitable for a nursing home. It is like a jail. Because they put us upstairs and they lock all the doors. The food is also not good.

What is it like upstairs?

Separate rooms are there. Many patients are there. It is not suitable to call it a nursing home.

What sort of treatment do you get?

The treatment is good. Very good. But we have to live upstairs and it makes pressure on your heart, to live inside this. It is like a jail.

What is your day like here, the routine, starting in the morning?

First they give the breakfast here. Then they bring all the patients downstairs to take a bath. Then they take them upstairs. Then they bring them downstairs again for eating. They give tea, and some *tiffin* to eat. Then at 9.30 dinner. The quality is very bad of course. The quality is bad and the living conditions are bad. It feels like a jail.

What are your fellow patients like?

Some of them are out of mind. Some are good.

Why are they out of mind?

Some of them are mad.

Why did they come here?

They came here. They had mental problems and all.

How did you used to live before this?

Before this I lived very well. In my house, I took nice kinds of food. I went to movie halls.

If you were totally free, what would you do now?

I would control myself. I would live in controlled manner. And I'd always be in contact with the divine.

The distressed husband. The third young man I met that day was from Basirhat and had been very violent. Dr Basu told me he had financial problems, had recently married and experienced erectile dysfunction. He had repeatedly tried to kill himself by hanging. When we visited the nursing home, the suicidal man was brought in. He could barely walk, and two attendants supported him on each side. He was shaking, and his face was lop-sided. His arms shook uncontrollably, and his tongue moved oddly outside his lips. His hands were frozen and he shivered, uncontrollably. None of the medication was working so the psychiatrist decided to give ECT. He rarely gave this form of treatment, perhaps only once a year, when all else failed. However, the following morning the man tried to strangle himself again, was stopped by another inmate who couldn't sleep, but who got badly bitten. The patient was under observation throughout the day and night. He responded well to the ECT, but had side effects from the drugs, so a cardiologist was brought in to check his heart. The staff were becoming tired watching over him, so the doctor ordered him to be restrained temporarily in order to give them a rest, so they could look after other patients.

The psychiatrist suggested calling in the family priest, since sometimes if they said a prayer for the dead, it would help lift any discarnate entities resting with a person. The following day the man's two brothers arrived. The doctor told them what had happened, said his medicines were having little effect, and there were side effects. He said they could change doctors if they wanted, and told them how their brother was determined to kill himself. When the brothers went to visit the Nursing Home, he tried to kill himself in front of them. The brothers mentioned an occultist who had told them there had been two suicides near his home, which were probably affecting him: one man had killed himself by poison, the other by hanging. The occultist thought the spirits of those two people who had killed themselves were over-shadowing the doctor's patient. The brothers performed a prayer to Kali on his behalf, and the psychiatrist also asked the astrologer SriRam to perform a prayer ritual for the man.

The doctor said: '*the planets affect my patient's well being: on the day of the dark moon (no moon day), many people try to kill themselves. I have lots of cases of attempted suicide on the days of no moon and full moon.*' In this case, the psychiatrist perceived the following treatments as necessary: medication, ECT (Electroconvulsive therapy), physical restraint, accompanied by prayers to the goddess Kali, and releasing of any attached spirits of the dead. He also mentioned the influence of the moon on patients.

The sign writer. While we were there at the clinic I was invited to interview Mohammad, a young man the Muslim cleric had first sent to the psychiatrist 10 years earlier. The doctor's wife translated. Mohammad was a calm, confident young man in his 30's, who had been visiting the cleric since he was a 10 year old child. He explained what caused his first upset that had triggered his distress. His elder sister was overshadowed (possessed) by a *djinn* (genie, spirit being) who was always with her, but didn't do her any harm, although it did make her go unconscious and talk to herself. The *djinn* became upset with him when he quarrelled with his sister, since this interfered with its being 'blissed out upon her', and it threatened to frighten him. The first time he had an encounter with the *djinn*, it took the shape of his mother: he was scared, had an attack and 'lost his balance'.

Whenever he had attacks he was taken to the Molovi, Haji Saheb, who gave him charms (*taviz*). He wore them around his neck, on his forearm, and around his waist. These would have a calming effect for several months, and then he was supposed to renew them for 'recharging'. "*There is a specific time period during which the taviiz works, and you have to replace it. That is categorical.*" But the journey cost a lot of money and so they didn't always go to recharge the charm, even if his condition became aggravated.

"*Although the Haji doesn't demand any money, it doesn't feel very good to go there and take everything free of charge.*"

The doctor's wife explained what happened next. "*On one such occasion he was brought to Dr Basu. He was chained, absolutely he was chained (with his arms crossed and his legs held together). When you are violent all your limbs are chained. His arms and legs were crossed and chained. He was in a terrible condition. The villagers pooled some money. They volunteered: they came forward and brought him to Dr Basu in that state. He was around 23 years old. It took 10 to 12 villagers to take him into town. He was violent and that is the reason he was chained. He did not walk to the chamber. They carried him on a van rickshaw. That is a bicycle, with a cart behind on two wheels. That is how he was brought to the chamber at Basirhat.*"

Dr Basu gave him an injection, and some medicines to take orally, and after some time his sleep pattern was restored. Mohammad explained about the combination of conditions that triggered the attack. He had been using the *taviiz* for around 12 years by then. He was 22 years old, in financial crisis, and the frequent 'occurrences' meant that he could not study, so he and his family had to live on charity. His father had died many years earlier in the 1980's, and to pay debts to relatives he was allowing them to use his father's land. Gradually he regained his strength. He was still on medicines, but on a dramatically reduced dose. Dr Basu suggested he didn't take any addictive material, even tea or betel nut, and he followed this. He used to take 6 to 7 pills a day and this was reduced to a maintenance dose of one. He hadn't had a relapse since he was 24, and now he was happily married with three young children, and worked as a sign writer.

During the interview Mohammad wanted to know why I had only been asking about the hard times he had experienced. "*You have been asking about his difficulties. Now the life he is living, he is so happy. He looks so happy. He wants you to understand that he is happy. He writes for a business and that is his only form of income. He is happily married and has a family. He has 3 children, two sons and a daughter. The villagers who brought him to see Dr Basu are jubilant."* He had tried many jobs, but when he tried writing, people found he wrote very clearly, and they started to give him books to read. *"Now he helps other people write letters, and he paints shop advertising signs. And in cinemas, where there are films showing, he writes the advertisements that are seen on the screen."* On our journey home, one of Mohammad's painted signs was pointed out: a pink lobster and pink prawns on a board outside a fishery. It was a fine painting.

Later Dr Basu commented: *"Mohammad has bipolar disorder. I have seen him twice in manic states, extremely violent, and chained. He was so poor he had to be treated on an outpatient basis, yet he responded dramatically. He was put on lithium but he always took a lower dose than prescribed, because of lack of money. However he has remained stable for ten years or more. In spite of his illness and medicines, he has continued to steadily draw signboards. Because of his intense faith in God and his doctor, he has managed to keep himself steady in spite of taking maintenance medication at a lower dose than prescribed."*

SUMMARY

I was grateful Dr Basu had given me the opportunity to speak with 25 of his patients, and that he, or his wife, or a former patient had translated. I understand the restrictions of having close people do translation and the subsequent potential 'filtering' of information that might occur. But that was how it was. It was interesting most patients I interviewed were Hindu, and in the (paid) nursing home, inpatients seemed to be of a particular caste, though privately Dr Basu was renowned for seeing anyone, whether or not they could pay.

I had tried years ago while I was in London, to see if I could conduct research into mental health service-user perspective, but I was only allowed to talk to former patients who were outside the psychiatric system. In Kolkata, I'd learnt that the consultation process was for the individual sufferer and for the family. The carers were included. It was interesting to realise that referrals were contemporaneous between professionals with skills that bridged medical, traditional occult and complementary practices. Some patients travelled hundreds of miles to see a good practitioner: they believed in the pharmacology and the spiritual treatments. It seemed that both doctor and patients believed in recovery, and worked towards that.

Temple practices and rituals on the one hand were seen as very useful, on the other might tip a person over the edge. There was a link made between spiritual experience and psychosis. I discovered that it was normal to consider the influence of spirits of the dead, djinn, and past lives, and the role of prayer seemed to be important, if not essential in some cases. In the following chapter I explore more about peoples' beliefs and explanations for the causes of their symptoms.

Chapter Four

PATIENTS' PERSPECTIVES AND CULTURAL INTERPRETATIONS

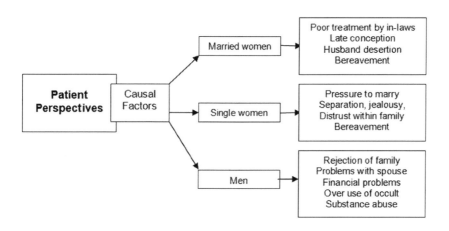

In this chapter I explore patient perspectives: beliefs informants had about the causes and triggers of their mental distress. I divided data from people I interviewed into three groups: married women; single women; and men. Although these three groups had theories of illness causation in common, there were other social triggers that appeared specific to certain groups. For example, married women may experience poor treatment by their in-laws, perhaps due to not being able to conceive, or they may be deserted by the husband. Single women may experience severe distress due to pressure to marry, or separation from their fiancé, or for reasons of jealousy or distrust. Men may have problems with their spouse, or with their financial affairs. There may be substance abuse, or 'over use' of occult practices which tip them into psychosis. All groups suffered in common as a result of bereavement or witnessing death. I present cultural interpretations suggested by different practitioners in Part Three, chapters 8 and 9.

During interviews, very few patients said they had been to any outside diagnostician, such as a priest or a healer. Perhaps they hadn't, or perhaps I was asking the wrong question in the wrong location. After all, who would admit to such things in psychiatrist's surgery? However some people did. I noticed a difference was expressed between the triggers for married and single women and for men, and so I have presented the data according to those categories.

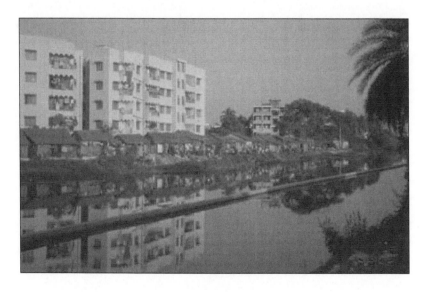

Kolkata waterways

Causal Factors: identified by Dr Basu's patients

Many of the patients I spoke to believed that the trigger for their mental distress came from the material world, from social, financial or relationships issues.

Married women. There were more marked differences between married and single women, and men in general. The main trigger for mental distress leading to disorder in the married women I spoke to was inconsiderate or poor treatment from their husband's family. On marriage women usually joined their husband's extended family, perhaps in a different village, town or region away from their own parental home. In some homes they were treated as domestic servants and they received little or no affection from the husband's family. The women felt poorly acknowledged and had no one to relate to, or share their feelings with. This meant some kept all their emotions bottled up, and became ill. Gradually as the husband's brothers married, new women would come into the household to help out with chores. Also their husband's sisters would marry and move out, and older women became frail and died, then as dynamics changed domestic conditions resolved.

CHART NO. 4.1
CAUSAL FACTORS WHICH TRIGGER MENTAL DISTRESS
(according to interviews with married female patients)

MARRIED WOMEN
- Poor treatment by in-laws
- Lack of love received from in-laws
- Bearing a child some years after marriage (i.e. late)
- Depression after the child's birth
- Desertion by husband
- Extra marital relationships (of self or spouse)
- Death of a relative, bereavement
- Experiencing presence of a deceased relative
- Love marriage to a poorer man, & parental refusal to pay dowry
- Having seen a suicide or unnatural death
- Hearing sounds in the head, and hallucinations

The stress that resulted from patrilocal residence for some women was exacerbated if a wife did not conceive. One 42 year old woman was married for seven years before she gave birth to a healthy baby. *"They were some problems. My school results were poor and this made me very upset, and I was suffering from that. After seven years of marriage I got my child. This long period. I really had a problem. I always thought, 'when will I get a child? Will I get child?' It gave me pain. I had to do only domestic jobs, as I had no qualifications and could not get any job. And in the family I had to do all the domestic jobs, and I had no child. So I was very depressed. I felt very bored. These thoughts made me a patient."*

Other women were upset because their in-laws refused to allow them to take a professional job outside marriage. Depression resulting from childbirth was another influence on a wife's health. This could be post-partum depression, or caused by frailty due to being forced back into domestic work too soon without adequate time to recover. [Usually women preferred to return to their parental household to give birth, and then went back to their husband's family several months later.]

One woman had been deserted by her husband, and was forced to return to her father's household. Her father subsequently remarried and she was treated badly by his new spouse. In addition, due to her mental state, her child was removed from her care and placed in a boarding school. In contrast another woman from a wealthy family decided upon a love marriage, and this meant she received no dowry. This caused problems since her parents refused to help financially to keep her in the style she was accustomed. She engaged in an extra-marital relationship, which although her husband forgave, she thought about it constantly. These things disturbed her so much she became suicidal.

Women who had lost a loved one found the bereavement hard to bear. Although one woman (SR, no.23) had problems from her husband's family, she'd had mental difficulties since she had been a child. She saw a murder then and had fits since that time. She was still grieving the death of her father, some three years earlier. She had repeated tried to kill herself by walking on railway lines at night, and hoarding pills so she could overdose. She explained: *"A Bengali joint family is a typical one. So I was mentally tortured, I couldn't express my feelings. They forced me to do this work and that work, what the doctor has told me not to do. I couldn't tell anyone. I cannot tell my mum and dad also. They will get hurt. My husband cannot say anything because he is the youngest in the family."*

"Three years ago my father expired. He was the closest one for me. He did everything for me. And that shock I couldn't tolerate. I can always feel my father is blessing me… I told my mum that I could feel my father's fingers. His fingers were bony. I could feel him patting my head. I told my mum, and my mum used to shout, 'stop thinking about your father'. She used to tell me, 'you are creating problems for his soul. He cannot go up'. My mum used to tell me. She used to scold me, 'stop crying for your father'…."

"My father in law is 89, and my mother in law is 82 years old. Sometimes I'd tell my husband that I am feeling jealous of him because you are having your father and mother, and I have lost my father. And he started laughing: 'He came, he passed away, and when their time comes, they will also pass away'."

"Still now my husband goes on talking to me. Saying 'what are you thinking?', I don't like to share anything with him. He is a very caring husband, very caring, very helpful. He took me here. He is always by my side. I am thinking that he is spending so much money on me. He is coming down to the doctor. He is paying for the medicine. It is all so upsetting. I am not giving him anything in life. He is just caring for me like a child. He is caring for me like my father also. He used to give me pills. He used to lie me down. He has to check my medicines and give me food. He used to take me out. He does so much for me. He is telling me, everyone is telling me, 'your presence is a real support for him'. I don't want to eat anything. I don't want to go anywhere. I don't want to put any new clothes. He is forcing me to put new dresses and to come out. He said 'let us go to our relative's house'. We have a long marriage."

This patient's husband was very supportive and very sincere in getting her treated. Dr Basu stressed that this support was critical for the well being of his married female patients (see treatment strategies below).

Single female patients. Single women were brought to the doctor's clinic either by their mothers alone, or by their mothers and sisters, or by both parents. One student arrived with her parents and both set of grandparents. All attended the 'individual' consultation. The factors that influenced single women and appeared to be triggers for their disorders were due to marriage: either through calling off a marriage, or separation from a boyfriend or fiancé. One girl became jealous of her lover, after seeing him get out of an auto-rickshaw with a friend, and called off the wedding. Pressure to marry caused additional strain, particularly if the girl was the oldest in her family and her sisters could not marry until she did. *"According to our Indian families in west Bengal, I have to marry first, then my younger sister can get her chance. So I'm in a dilemma."* Women and girls also feel a strain if they are unmarried while their peer group of relatives and friends are already married. Girls who had poor school results, experienced distress, since this meant they could not progress to a job, or have a career they wanted. It affected their self-esteem.

Loss or separation from a potential marriage suitor can be an underlying factor of distress. One girl studying away from home fell pregnant, and was upset after her lover insisted she had an abortion. She had been very happy when she fell pregnant. But her boyfriend was not. *"I felt so happy. I told him over the phone and he didn't react, then he telephoned me after my class and said 'get aborted'. I was so shocked. I thought OK, I'll tell my parents and he'll tell his parents and we will get married. And he said 'no I can't do that. I am not prepared to get married or be a father. Get aborted'. I said 'no I won't', and he said 'if you won't then I'll commit suicide'. He was blackmailing me...."*

CHART NO. 4.2
CAUSAL FACTORS WHICH TRIGGER MENTAL DISTRESS
(according to interviews with single female patients)

SINGLE WOMEN

○ MARRIAGE

- ❖ Calling off a marriage
- ❖ Pressure on self, as oldest child, to marry
- ❖ Strain of being an unmarried girl/woman
- ❖ jealous of fiancé
- ❖ Loss or separation from boyfriend or lover

○ LOSS

- ❖ Abortion
- ❖ Death of a relative, bereavement
- ❖ Having seen a suicide or unnatural death
- ❖ Being from a refugee family
- ❖ Poor academic qualifications

○ PROBLEMS WITH THEIR FAMILY

- ❖ Distrust of father, parents,
- ❖ Jealousy of sibling,
- ❖ Not being believed by family

○ PROBLEMS WITH RELATIONSHIP

- ❖ Unwanted male attention
- ❖ Problems with the neighbours

This patient had chosen to see the psychiatrist of her own free will since her depression and inability to work was frustrating her ambitions. *"Before coming here I was about to commit suicide... I used to think about how I would die... And I thought 'no, my parents are divorced and my sister got married two years back and my mother she is so lonely'. Thank God I had this much capacity to think about my mother. Otherwise I would have died. I was on the verge."*

The final influence for mental disorder in unmarried girls was problems concerned with relationship, whether of their own family, or from neighbours. One 22 year old girl was brought in since she had begun to distrust her father and this distressed her terribly. A very bright engineering student, she had received unwanted attentions from a married male neighbour, who had made improper suggestions to her, followed her and threatened rape.

She felt as if her father was colluding with this man to prostitute her, and she was distraught no one in the family believed her story. *"I feel very tense. I can't make anyone believe that I am right. Everyone is trying to prove that I am mad. I don't think I am mad. I am perfectly all right. Do you think I am mad?"* I asked her how she might resolve this situation with her family, and then continue with her studies. *"I am going to pretend to be normal. I am going to react normally. I have to say sorry to everyone. I am going to suppress the whole feelings. I can behave normally. Of course this will give a very good impression. I will try to concentrate on my studies. What to do? This is going to create a big impression on my mind and I am not going to forget it. A cat is going to come out of the bag someday, somehow. This is an incident. There is an occurrence and there is a problem. I am sure of it. I have to say 'forgive me, I had thought something wrong. I am sorry for the whole incident. I have reacted very violently'. Publicly, in front of everyone, I say this."*

Whose Problem? I asked Dr Basu to tell me whose problem it was when a wife had mental health problems. I wanted to know whether there were any other cultural differences. The previous week he mentioned the case of a husband who believed his wife's psychiatric problems were the responsibility of her parents. He explained about the notion of the self and the individual: *"In India, the 'self' is an extended social self, not individualistic as in the West. While this has an adaptive value in situations where social support plays an important role, it has a maladaptive value when a husband* *shifts responsibility for his wife's treatment onto his wife's parents. However, the impact of globalisation means the value of individualism is percolating here in the upper strata of society."*

He continued *"Indian society is very pluralistic. There are many levels of culture and society. So streaks of individualism are now manifesting in the middle and upper classes. But in the lower social classes, individualism has not got that hold. So when women suffer psychiatric problems, then the husbands think their wife's parental family are responsible for that, and they should bear the cost and take responsibility for the treatment. In the upper stratum of society, individualism gains more momentum, then the man will not accuse the woman in this way."*

"Mental illness is different from physical body illness. Physical ailments like chronic tuberculosis, men might expect the parental family to take some responsibility, some liability, but with psychiatric disorders some lower classes think the wife's parents should accept liability. This is a common occurrence in a male dominated society, where individualism has not gathered momentum. It is particularly so in the case of psychiatry although not for biological disorders of the body."

Dr Basu told me about one woman interviewed, whose husband was initially non-cooperative, because he originally thought the treatment for his wife's psychiatric problems was the liability of his wife's parents. He said there were particular difficulties for young women and girls with psychiatric problems, because they embodied honour and shame for their families. Such shame did not extend so much to men with psychiatric problems.

Male Patients. Men experienced a slightly different range of influences, which affected their mental health. Some were similar to women such as from loss, like a fiancé calling off their marriage, divorce, the death or a relative, or due to being from a refugee family. Others were affected by having seen a suicide or an unnatural death. One man was affected by the birth of his sister's handicapped baby, and her subsequent mistreatment by her in-laws. A social worker translated: *"His older sister, she gave birth to a handicapped baby three months ago. The baby is not having both her hands, so he was very tense about it, and he saw his mother crying about it. He is disturbed, that the baby is born handicapped... About his mother-in-law, she is not very good. His sister should have proper rest, but their mother in law makes her work, to wash dishes, and do the regular work of the family. It is hard for her. He thinks this will affect his sister and he feels his sister should have rest, and not do all the work. He feels it will adversely affect his sister's life and maybe she will die."*

Men also had problems with their families. This might be distrust of their parents, or having quarrels with relatives. One man felt his sister was not paying adequate attention to their sick father, and after a quarrel he renounced his family and did not take up his inheritance. Born to the *kayestu* or royal caste, another man rejected his family's values, and lived a politicised life until drugs and drink got the better of him, and he ended up in the gutter. In contrast, a 16 year old boy in the Nursing home appeared to detest his father's lowly occupation as a seller of undergarments, and had shown violence towards his mother. Thus both too much wealth and too much poverty could be influences that led to mental disorder.

CHART NO.4.3
CAUSAL FACTORS WHICH TRIGGER MENTAL DISTRESS
(according to interviews with male patients)

MALE PATIENTS (SINGLE AND MARRIED)

○ **LOSS**
  ❖ Of a girlfriend, calling off a marriage
  ❖ Birth of married sister's handicapped baby, and her subsequent mistreatment by in-laws
  ❖ Divorce
  ❖ Death of a relative, bereavement
  ❖ Having seen a suicide or unnatural death
  ❖ Being from a refugee family

○ **PROBLEMS WITH FAMILY**
  ❖ Distrust of parents, quarrels with relatives
  ❖ Renunciation of family after quarrels
  ❖ Refusal by siblings to share inheritance
  ❖ Rejection of family situation (too much wealth)
  ❖ Detest family social standing (too much poverty)
  ❖ Problems with spouse
    • Erectile dysfunction
    • Domestic problems

○ **FINANCIAL PROBLEMS, CRISES**
○ **SUCCESS – RECEIVED A DEGREE, OVER-HAPPY**
○ **EXISTENTIAL PAIN (OF BEING)**
○ **OVER USE OF OCCULT POWERS & CLAIRVOYANCE**
○ **OVER USE OF OCCULT RITUALS**
○ **INGESTING HARMFUL SUBSTANCES GIVEN BY AN OCCULTIST**
○ **ATTACKED BY A DJINN WHO HAD OVERSHADOWED SISTER**
○ **FAILURE TO RECHARGE A CHARM (TAVIZ) GIVEN BY PIR (MUSLIM HOLY MAN)**
○ **MULTIPLE SUBSTANCE ABUSE**

Financial problems created stress for mental disorder as did erectile dysfunction for one married man, and domestic quarrels for another who was a librarian. One man in his late 30's was a taxi driver from the schedule caste, who developed a disorder from too much happiness. He became overjoyed when he achieved his LLB law exam, had grandiose ideas, then burnt out and had a break down. He came to Dr Basu's notice, and was put in the nursing home. In contrast another young man experienced existential pain of being incarnate on earth where inhabitants did not respect the resources of the planet.

In addition to above mentioned triggers, there were occult reasons given for mental disturbance. For example Mohammad was attacked by djinn who had overshadowed his sister. His failure to re-energise the amulet *(taviz)* given to him by a Muslim holy man reduced his protection, and he experienced mental disorder again.

Then there was the case of SriRam, who had manic attacks whenever he did too much intuitive astrological work. He became strained when he over used his occult and clairvoyant powers. He had undertaken rituals at one temple, where he meditated on corpses. As part of his initiation with a tantric priest he had ingested substances, which he felt had affected his well-being. These included ashes from a cremated corpse and the brain of a dead owl. [Ingesting ashes from a deceased relative is not unusual in India[38], as well as giving ashes to a river[39], so the soul is released and can travel onwards. Consumption of ashes is a sacred ritual].

There were other cases of men like Ariram who over consumed more ordinary substances like 'brown sugar' (heroin), LSD, and alcohol. Even while working at the doctor's clinic on rehabilitation, Ariram had a tendency to scan rooms for any sedatives within his reach and 'pop' them, which made him rather drowsy. He had refined features and sluggish eyes, and was often very self tranquillised. When he came off his medication his thinking became illogical, whereas the doctor said, on medication he was calm and appeared quiet and immaculately well spoken, and articulate.

Changing Cultural Interpretations of Mental Distress

The psychiatrist explained over the decades, the diagnoses he made for his patients' conditions appeared to change so that they did not neatly fit the DSM. *"Twenty years ago we used to differentiate clear-cut paranoid and depressive patients. Now gradually in India, we see an equal mixture of paranoid and depressive components in patients under stress, who are otherwise not disorganised or schizophrenic, not so delusional to be classed solely under delusional disorder, and not solely depressed, so that they can be called endogenous depression, and their illnesses do not run a cyclical course to be labelled as bipolar disorder or cyclical psychosis. They do not fit in with other classical paradigms. Perhaps this is an indication of changing cultural norms, urbanisation, loss of cultural identity."*

There were other interpretations of his patients' conditions, which were not considered 'normal' within western psychiatry. When speaking about a case of one young man in a locked nursing home, he suggested that past life therapy might throw some light on his condition, to help understand his behaviour. He said the man had an identity crisis and was a misfit within his social class. Other patient's conditions equally did not fit neatly into western models. *"This man has a borderline personality disorder with a history of multiple substance abuse and deviancy, and streaks of schizoid thoughts. His diagnosis does not fit into classical ICD10 and DSM IV grooves, and we have found that a holistic approach was more suited."*

Some patients seemed to maintain a good state of health, even though taking a lower dose of medication. Dr Basu pointed out *"W.H.O. has written that the prognosis of schizophrenia is much better in India, so they always tell us that the prognosis is better in countries like Egypt, India, and China. These they refer to as Third World Countries, but actually we should be considered as Ancient Cultures."*

"People should ask 'why do these countries have a better prognosis'? And with a better prognosis, that means you do not have to carry that label all along, like for example the taxi driver HS. He had an episode, then for the last ten years he hasn't had anything, and I'm still giving him a low dose due to my modern European training, as I do not want to take any risks. If I did not have that European training I would not have given him so much medication. It is because of that, that I am still giving him medication. But in between he has been composed, and sober, and he doesn't carry any stigma of that manic episode which occurred once."

I asked Dr Basu to confirm what he was saying, that although many of his patients had an episode once or twice, they weren't considered mentally ill by those around them. He said the occurrence was seen as an episode of something that happened, but it wasn't a label they had for life. *"When something happens, it is more likely to be considered to do with their situation, their subtle senses, or with possession states, so they don't have to carry stigma. This makes a huge difference. The label is very heavy. I think we are unnecessarily spending too much energy on labelling diseases, especially psychiatric diseases."*

Dr Basu appeared to be fed up with western cultural projections and assumptions. *"Western psychiatrists say our depression in India is somatised more, especially through abdominal symptoms. We don't have a proper terminology for depression as a disease as you have in other languages. Depression may be a mood, or a symptom, but it may also be a disease. But depression as a disease doesn't have any translation equivalent as a Sanskrit word."*

"What we have are terms that qualify depression as a mood. We somatise depression, it doesn't usually come as 'blues', like you have in the west, but it usually comes through somatic symptoms, abdominal symptoms. And that is acceptable in our culture. It is not be because our cultural level is lower than in the west, which was the old thinking, or that our language or our culture was deficient, but because it is acceptable. Somatisation is very acceptable in our culture. That removes the stigma." He continued *"We recognise somatisation as a form of depression, that is a group of disorders that are linked with depression, and they respond to antidepressants for us."*

The psychiatrist also considered that religious assumptions influenced allocation of symptoms to a particular disorder, and that social influences resulted in change through time. *"I think that cultural differences have a very important role to play, for example at one time guilt was an important symptom of depression in the west. Now we see interesting changes, that guilt in the west is being replaced by low self-esteem. In India guilt was never a highly important symptom of depression. This is mainly because of the difference in cultural attitudes towards guilt. In the West, because of Christianity, man is considered to be a sinner, but here in India we say 'amrita shiyaputra', a human being is the son of immortality."*

SUMMARY

It seemed as if in India, fundamental belief systems about the nature of human existence influenced both clinicians' diagnosis of mental ill health and treatment, and their patients' acceptance of diagnosis and responses to treatment. We were introduced to different cultural notions of 'individual' and 'self'.

The mundane causal factors for triggers of distress for single women were jealousy, mistrust, pressure to marry or separation from fiancé, or loss due to bereavement (which was common to many patients). Married women had some different triggers including delayed conception, poor treatment from husband's family, and desertion. For men there were other factors such as financial problems, rejection, poor relationship with spouse, and substance abuse.

Triggers for mental distress came from the material world, with social, financial or relationship concerns. However, there were also some occult explanations for triggers, including being attacked by djinn, failure to power-up prophylactic charms, witnessing an unnatural death, and over-use of occult rituals. In Section Three I consider in more detail mundane and esoteric explanatory models (Chapters 8 and 9).

As well as biological, psychological factors and bereavement, practitioners suggested causal factors included planetary influences, effects of karma from a previous existence, and spirit possession. Practitioners were aware of the importance of spiritual matters, like different levels of consciousness, and soul energy. The psychiatrist thought his diagnoses did not always fit the

DSM manual, and although he considered stigma and guilt western concepts, South Asian citizens in UK may feel it is a reality. The concept of women embodying shame more than men with mental distress seems to be ubiquitous. Somatisation of symptoms of distress seemed normal in India, as did the notion of recovery from distress.

In Part Two I describe a variety of treatments observed during fieldwork. Covered in three chapters, these include: pharmacology, and remedies like those made from flowers; pilgrimage to sacred places to address mental distress; and finally visits to spiritual places to ensure mental peace.

PART TWO

TREATMENT STRATEGIES

Treatment Strategies

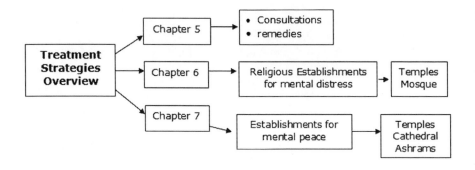

Treatment strategies from a variety of healing modalities

This section is divided into three chapters. In the first (chapter 5), I present the remedies for mental health, used by the medical and complementary practitioners I interviewed. In Chapter 6, I set out a selection of religious establishments renowned for their treatment of the mentally distressed. In Chapter 7, I cover spiritual organisations, which pilgrims visit in order to achieve mental peace. Overleaf there is a chart listing the range of treatment strategies used.

CHART NO. 5.1
RANGE OF TREATMENT STRATEGIES
According to practitioners, accessed by their patients singly, sequentially, or contemporaneously

CONSULTATION:

○ One or more physician or psychiatrist
  ❖ Western pharmacology, ECT, restraint
  ❖ Housed in locked nursing home, government asylum
○ Astrologers or palm readers
○ Palm Leaf Oracles
○ Traditional healers (*oja*) or traditional teachers (*gurus*)
○ Referrals between different types of practitioner

REMEDIES FOR HEALING

○ Herbal remedy correlated with planets, and earth, air, fire, water
○ Homoeopathic remedies
○ Flower remedies
○ Acupuncture
○ Counselling

RELIGIOUS ACTIVITIES

○ Prayer or initiating contact with the Divine
○ Religious cleansing rituals (temple, mosque, church)
○ Taking in vibrations of a deity or saint at a shrine
○ Making a pilgrimage or tour
○ Prayer, devotion, sacrifice
○ Chanting and saying of *mantras*
○ Use of smouldering camphor & incense
○ Wearing of amulets, charms, sacred threads
○ Propitiation of deities, planets, trees, land areas, water sources

ENVIRONMENT, MODIFIED LOCATION

○ Travel to other areas, living with different family members
○ Modified architecture, compound walls, colours, design
○ Healing through being in psychiatrist's waiting room & conferring with others in a similar situation.

Chapter Five

REMEDIES AND PHYSICIANS

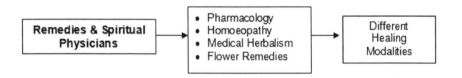

| Remedies & Spiritual Physicians | → | • Pharmacology
• Homoeopathy
• Medical Herbalism
• Flower Remedies | → | Different Healing Modalities |

Remedies used by Medical and Complementary Practitioners

In the previous chapters we learnt people consulted with medical, religious, and complementary therapy practitioners to enhance their mental well being. As a researcher, I wanted to understand how practitioners explained the relationship between bio-medicine and other remedies.

This chapter is structured around my interviews with practitioners, who used remedies to address mental ill health: an Indian psychiatrist, who incorporated western pharmacology with spiritual strategies; a senior homoeopath; a former surgeon who practiced homoeopathy; a medical herbalist who told me remedies offered to patients were correlated to the planets;

and an American psychiatrist from Harvard who used flower essences.

I discovered flower remedies were used by a couple of psychiatrists alongside their pharmacological treatments, together with acupuncture and some counselling at the clinic in Calcutta. Medical practitioners suggested a range of complementary and alternative remedies to treat patients with mental illness including the participation in worship and healing rituals in temples.

The Psychiatrist:
Pharmacology and Religious Strategies

Dr Basu's treatment strategies for patients included psychiatric pharmacology, counselling, social interventions, compulsory restraint in a locked nursing home, and ECTs in extreme cases. Government asylums were available for patients with acute disorders, who could not afford the private nursing home. However Dr Basu waived his fees for poorer clients, or negotiated that they pay only for food and lodging. If Dr Basu felt his treatment was not working, he would invite the patient's relatives in for a chat. He would explain the situation to them, and advise them that they could take the patient to another psychiatrist if they wanted to. At the clinic, Dr Basu considered supporting the patient to focus on spiritual matters ameliorated their disorders, and restored self-esteem.

The psychiatrist was aware some patients had visited occultists and traditional healers both before and during their treatments with him, and he was sensitive to this, as can be seen by the visit to the Muslim cleric in Chapter Two. Often he would suggest patients undertook religious activities or ritual practices as part of their treatment regime. He was sceptical of those who charged for such advice, for he felt it was common sense to use smouldering incense and burning camphor to cleanse a person, place, or atmosphere, of its energies, in order to promote well being.

Sometimes the psychiatrist suggested a patient undertake a career change or choose a new line of study more in keeping with their own beliefs or situation (patient no.12 AB). He said one man (no.8 NB) had endogenous depression due to an existential crisis. *"He is on amitryptoline, but he requires intensive counselling. He himself reads anything and knows the limitations of a cognitive approach, hence we always deal with him in a holistic way trying to help him in personal growth, trying to expand his intellectual horizons. This does not per se reduce his depression, but it gives him sustenance to battle with life. He especially appreciates not being treated as a patient."*

Dr Basu's perception of his treatment strategies was clear. His aim was always to stabilise his patients by whatever means required, and then use the lowest possible dose of medication to maintain this. His intention was to allow a dose low enough to permit the patient to carry on with his or her daily life, to encourage their intuitive abilities (e.g. SriRam), their creative music abilities (e.g. Ariram, M, SC), or their creative painting skills (e.g. Mohammed). A list of treatment strategies is presented in Chart 5.1.

Psychiatric Diagnoses

The psychiatrist's diagnoses given to patients are summarised in the chart below (no.5.2) together with the pharmacological treatments. I cannot comment on either of these since I do not have a background in psychiatry and am not familiar with the diagnostic symptoms, treatment regimes, nor with the drugs prescribed. The additional treatments tried by patients contemporaneously with psychiatric pharmacology are summarised in the final column of the chart. The knowledge base for diagnosis Dr Basu worked from was western psychiatry, plus his personal sensitivity due to the addition of prayer and divine intervention of the Mother and Sri Aurobindo[40].

Dr Basu mentioned sometimes his diagnoses of patients fell outside the W.H.O. criteria, and outside the DSM criteria. I wondered how this affected a patient's spiritual well-being. *"In India we follow the W.H.O or the American DSM criteria. Psychiatrists should have two types of classification systems: one should be a public classificatory system, which is necessary for having a common denominator. In this way we can keep records of comparable notes, and have a common basis of knowledge. But side by side one should also have a private classification system. So I always carry two classificatory systems: the public for official work, and the other private system."*

"In that way I can see people at different levels of consciousness, and I perceive the problems at different levels. If I see that someone's inner being is strong, then I'd give him or her less medicine. I try to bring out the spirit in them. And then I try to find out if a person is very sensitive about his soul energy. So the personality can be gathered around his soul energy. There are different dimensions."

Dr Basu said he thought that in India the prescription of low doses of psychiatric medication was due to cultural factors. *"Previously in India practitioners and clinicians used to think that because a westerner's average body weight was more, they required a higher dosage, whereas here in India, people respond to much lower doses than prescribed in western textbooks. This is always the case. At first we thought it was due to our lower body weight, but now we think it is because of our culture."*

"We believe in many lives, so a little improvement is accepted heartily. But in the western world, where you believe in one life, you believe you have to be better, completely better. So we think you require more medicines,

because you believe one life span is the only one given to you. Here because of our belief in many lives, we accept a little improvement. Of course this comment would be called unscientific by western standards..!"

Dr Basu explained that he intentionally gives patients *"less lithium than required (for maintenance medication), so as not thwart creativity. I personally use this approach, whenever a patient has a high degree of genuine creativity. I would always try not to thwart their talent by drugs hence I always give less quantity and keep such a subject under more intense surveillance (to detect any impending relapse at an early stage)."* At the clinic, he also considered that supporting the patient to focus on spiritual matters seemed to help ameliorate their disorders, and restore self-esteem.

CHART NO. 5.2.
PATIENTS DIAGNOSES, TREATMENT, & ALTERNATIVES

No.	Initials	Diagnosis	treatment	Additional treatments tried
1	SB	Manic depressive psychosis	Valproate, mood stabiliser	Prayer & temple rituals Works in clinic
2	AR	borderline personality disorder, multiple substance abuse, schizoid thoughts	lithium, carbamazapine and clozapine in low doses, respiridol	Poetry, music therapy, creative works, works in clinic
3	MSAM	bipolar disorder, manic states	Lithium	Faith in Allah, protective amulets for neck, forearm, waist, from Muslim cleric
4	AS	paranoid disorder (delusional disorder)	Compulsory restraint valproate and clozapine.	Spirituality
5	PD	grief reactive psychosis, with paranoid and manic elements, one post partum	Venlafaxine and lithium	Oja (traditional healer), rituals, mantras, charms
6	M	Depression, negative attitudes	behavioural counselling	Temple rituals, singing devotional songs
7	SC	bipolar disorder (Manic Depressive Psychosis)	Lithium	Creativity, classical music, composes & sings ragas
8	NB	endogenous depression	amitriptyline	Other doctors: CAT scan and EEG, psychoanalyst, change of career
9	KM	Depression, coexisting manic/ paranoid symptoms	(valpraote and trifluoperazine)	occult remedies: praying, burning camphor, stones charged with power
10	MS	bipolar disorder	Compulsory restraint	Past life therapies.?
11	HS	acute psychotic episode	Lithium, Compulsory restraint (formerly)	
12	AB	paranoid and depressive components	Olanzepine and ventafaxine	Training in a new discipline so he can work at home
13	MH	manic depressive psychosis	valproic acid	2 other doctors, supportive husband

No.	Initials	Diagnosis	treatment	Additional treatments tried
		CHART NO. 5.2. CONTINUED PART 2 **PATIENTS DIAGNOSES, TREATMENT, AND ALTERNATIVES**		
14	MS	disorder of impulse control, obsessive personality traits	'tablets'	
15	CB	brief reactive psychosis'		
16	MRS	'paranoid disorder' or 'delusional disorder'	Sleeping pills	Other doctors, Supportive husband, oja for protective amulet
17	RS	Paranoid, compulsive ritualistic behaviour.	Compulsory restraint, ECT (formerly), haloperidol and lithium, anti-depressants	no
18	SR	paranoid ideas, bulimic binges, impulsive behaviour	Clozapine SSRI	No, other psychiatrists
19	MS	Depressed, suicidal	light mood stabilisers and extensive counselling.	
20	KP	manic depression, obsessive compulsive paranoid ideas	clozapine, lithium, and clomipramine.	Other psychiatrists, ECTs
21	RP		Compulsory restraint, ECT	Prayer rituals, flower remedies
22	NS	disorder of impulse control obsessive traits in personality	lithium and clomipramine.	Supportive husband, Oja, amulets for arm & neck (one Hindu, one Muslim), mantras, temple prayers
23	SR	Psychogenic fits that is, pseudo seizures.	Ventafaxine and valproic acid	Other doctors, EEG epilepsy, Supportive husband
24	JS	paranoid, had strong organised delusions	Compulsory restraint (formerly) clozapine	
25	RN	Histrionic, psychopathic traits	mood stabiliser	

The Homoeopathic Physician:
Collaboration with Allopathy

I was interested to discover how physicians of homoeopathy regarded allopathic treatments for mental distress, and the kind of relationship they had with practitioners. Several homoeopath physicians considered allopathic medicine was marvellous for crisis and emergencies. It was excellent when a person's life needed saving, whereas homoeopathy effected a radical cure and worked more slowly and deeply.

One practitioner commented: *"Allopathic medicine has done something great. Allopathy in life saving emergencies, sometimes it has been very wonderful. For example allopathic medicine has developed systems that allow them to revive a person when they are physically in crisis. The person's life can be saved."* However a junior doctor sounded a note of caution as he felt that many Indian medical physicians had turned their back on traditional healing systems: *"I feel we forgot what we have in India, and we blindly turned towards the west for all things, while what we have to offer is much more in terms of our medical systems."*

Dr. Pachegaonkar, the Senior Homoeopath at the Medical Centre in Pondicherry, explained how allopathic medicine fitted in with the philosophy on which homoeopathy was based. He felt some allopathic doctors didn't understand the total picture of illness causation, of the human condition.

He explained: *"we do take assistance from allopathic physicians in certain areas. Basically the homoeopathic approach is that we enhance the healing ability of the patient through our remedies. Our remedies do not act directly with the disease pathology. Our medicines stimulate the healing force within, and then in turn the disease is eradicated. This is the principal of homoeopathy."*

"Sometimes what happens is a homeopathic kind of stimulation, which results in healing taking a long period for example over six months. If, within that time, the person succumbs to the disease pathology, then there is no point in a radical cure. Under such situations, especially when there is advanced pathology, we advocate palliative therapy, using allopathic methods. This might mean surgery or antibiotics, or even steroids as a life saving measure. But we are not trained in the application of these remedies, so when we recognise cases where palliation is needed, we take help from a good allopathic doctor.

Once the situation is palliated then we apply homoeopathic remedies for a more radical cure. For example in the case of renal calculus, we don't expect the body to expel a large stone. We take help from allopathic technology, where the stone is crushed and eliminated. At the same time we advocate homoeopathic treatment whereby the original tendency for the creation of stones is removed. So we work in collaboration. We complement each other."

However, he added: *"we don't get original or fresh cases. Unfortunately we get cases where people have been under allopathy for a number of years. Under these situations we have to taper off the dosage very cautiously because the person might have become drug dependant. Even if the original ailment is cured, the drug dependency is a problem. So we take help from the allopathic doctors in reducing the doses. It may take six months or two or three years."*

When Dr Pachegaonkar arrived in Pondicherry and came into contact with the philosophy of Sri Aurobindo and the Mother, he found it fitted well with homoeopathic philosophy. It seemed what Hahnemann said some 170 years earlier was very similar: the Mother and Sri Aurobindo described it in more spiritual ways, although they applied the principles in a practical manner. *"We have read the Organon since our college days, but now after going through the teachings of Mother and Sri Aurobindo, our vision is wider and deeper... Hahnemann used certain words like 'higher purpose of life'. Before, we didn't really understand it, but now we realise what it meant."*

He discovered he could relate homoeopathy to the planes of consciousness that Sri Aurobindo described: *"the awareness or comprehension, and then the application at every level, has been the phenomena which has set the criteria for homoeopathic prescriptions. Our understanding of the levels of consciousness has been much clearer after reading his philosophies."*

I was told this senior homoeopath had worked on some brilliant cases, which allopathic doctors had not been able to treat, and as a result of his homoeopathic cures he had become famous.

Dr Pachegoankar had considerable experience working in collaboration with allopathic doctors. He set up a rural medical college in his native place, and this was the first in rural India. He explained: *"medical staff at this rural college were very open and we used to work in collaboration. Under supervision of the experts in allopathy, we used to treat patients with homoeopathy.*

We used to choose diseases, which were not amenable to conventional allopathy, e.g. Psoriasis, skin disease, and rheumatoid arthritis.... The allopathic doctors would convince their patients that there was no treatment according to their medicine, and if the person was willing they would refer them to me. Sometimes the case would come directly to me and I would identify it and diagnose it based on my studies at medical college. So we were treating cases under supervision of allopathic experts and there were full medical records."

Dr Pachegaonkar gave one example of homoeopathic remedies offered to patients with mental health problems:

"When I started my practice, I was told not to treat cases of mental health." He was working in quite a small local area and if he failed to treat a case, it would become known and people would not trust his abilities. However during his second month at the clinic, a physician treating a woman with mental health problems had told her family that he could do nothing else for her, and she had to be admitted to the mental asylum. Her son, a teacher well known in the local community, did not want her to be admitted. Dr Pachegaonkar undertook multiple sittings with the patient and her family. Gradually the mother was cured by following the homoeopathic doctor's advice, and lived a further 18 years without symptoms. Dr Pachegoankar's senior colleague was Dr Mistry from Solapur.

The Surgeon:
Allopath and Homoeopath

There was one doctor I met at Pondicherry who had wide ranging interests in health, reality and existence, from different cultures all over the world. I felt a close connection with him: one year I went to Sri Aurobindo's room, as was the custom to celebrate my birthday. Dr Mistry and I had sat next to each other during this birthday meditation, but hadn't actually met before. Then we were introduced to each other shortly after at the Medical Centre in Pondicherry.

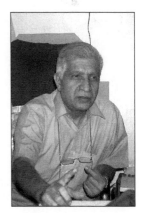

Dr Mistry

Dr Mistry was curious about other systems of belief and new paradigms. He studied physics, chemistry, and biology, and then specialised in medicine. In 1952 he entered a mainstream allopathic medical college in Puna, did his MBBS in 1957, and finished a Masters in Surgery in 1962. He settled in his home town of Solapur where he taught anatomy and anaesthesia at the allopathic medical college before switching to surgery. Today he is a practicing homoeopath and a follower of Sri Aurobindo.

I wondered what made Dr Mistry switch disciplines from allopathic medicine to homoeopathy. He explained: *"My first trigger was Sri Aurobindo's fondness for homoeopathy and his admiration for Hahnemann. Also I had read the lives of many masters by then, and most like Ram Krishna and Mahatma Gandhi, had very strong faith in homoeopathy. Finally, my father was an asthmatic, and when he went into a state I did not want to use steroids. So we brought him out somehow and he survived the last seven years of his life on homoeopathy.*

So from the age of 70 to 77 he was on pure homoeopathy. By that time I had read enough to treat him, and immediate family members, and most of the patients in the surgical hospital in my unit. I used to give homoeopathy to my operative cases, post-operative and pre-operative."

I asked how his allopathic medical colleagues responded to his preference for homoeopathy. *"There was a lot of resistance, especially from those colleagues who were rigid allopaths. They asked 'how can this man, who is teaching allopathy and mainstream medical studies, how can he give homoeopathy to his unit'? However, my bosses were all my patients, and they said 'OK, he is giving this treatment from his own pocket, and the government is not spending a single rupee. In fact he is saving the government hundreds and thousands of rupees because allopathic drugs are not being used. The patients are not complaining, so what harm is there?' However my colleagues tried really hard to make things difficult for me and there was some opposition. So I started up on my own. I left the college."*

Therapeutic Systems: Allopathy v. Homoeopathy.

I wanted to understand more about the relationship between homoeopathy and other medical systems. I asked Dr Mistry how homoeopathy functioned with spiritual aspects of health treatments. How did it work? *"Most of the alternative systems, they deal with certain aspects of energy levels. These include acupuncture and acupressure, which are based on subtle energy. Homoeopathy is one of the highest aspects, where the energy levels are so high, that they are unimaginable when you give a higher potency. We can see the shift of mainstream allopathic medicine towards the homoeopathic type of energy medicine, which others have been practising for hundreds of years. That is treating a person as a whole, and not by their parts. We progressively enter into subtle levels of energy."*

"Allopathy does not deal with the spiritual level: it is at the extreme edge of the spectrum of physicality. What allopathy has done so far is only one type of medication. It does not have a total overview that integrates the mind and emotional feeling at their depths, and all the structures and cells at their depths. Intelligence of consciousness comes when you transcend gross matter and move into subtle matter."

"What does the homoeopathic remedy do? It is a form of intelligence, a form of energy, a form of information, which Hahnemann discovered 250 years ago. At the far end of the spectrum, when you go into deeper and deeper levels of energy, and then from energy you have to go into consciousness. There is a stage where energy and consciousness are intermixed. The energy levels become more and more subtle, so that consciousness and energy become one."

Dr Mistry explained that allopathy dealt with physical matter, and homoeopathy and the others involved more subtle energies. I asked him how these related to something he mentioned earlier: shamanic treatments. "*The basic aspects of shamanism deal with forces, nature forces, occult forces, forces that are beyond the gross levels, which ultimately influence us all the time. If we are living in a unified world, in a unified cosmos, and all the other things are there, then shamanism has a role to play in an area in which mainstream medicine is not aware, for example in the area of spirit possession. Mainstream allopathic medicine is still uneasy: it cannot accept the involvement of discarnate energies that influence human illness and human health.*"

He explained to me about his perception of schizophrenia and epilepsy, which he said in each case, once the physical causes were eliminated from the diagnosis, then one had to address spiritual explanations. I wanted to understand what symptoms occurred, that were created by discarnate energies or spirits. He said: "*That is very difficult to answer, since there are so many types of energies that can influence a person. On the medical level for example take epilepsy and schizophrenia. There are so many aspects of schizophrenia that if you exclude the material level, a brain tumour, TB, or traumas, if you exclude material deep-set mind disorders, schizophrenia is to a great extent, from a spiritual point of view, involved with entities that are trying to influence human beings. They are energies. They are forces. They are intelligences, and they are discarnate.*"

"*You can remove forces by using shamanic techniques. You can even remove them by psychotherapy, or you can remove them using the protective influences of a good homoeopathic remedy. Even counselling or religious practices will help. For example, there are many situations in which one could give treatments for epilepsy. One can go on taking these throughout ones' life, and suffer the side effects, and maybe they are moderately useful in one's personal life. However, real epilepsies are definitely those, which are caused by outside forces, which we cannot see, because they are beyond our normal range of sensory perception. The shamans, occultists and*" *masters can see these things, and they take the necessary steps to remedy them."*

Therapeutic Systems: Integration or separation?

Given Dr Mistry's interest in other paradigms of reality, I asked whether he would like the therapeutic techniques of allopathic medicine and complementary practices to be integrated. He told me that each kind of healing practice should be clear about its own boundaries: "w*e are already moving towards a sort of integration, though integration does not necessarily mean that each accepts the other. I feel integration is to some extent allowing others to be as they are. I feel that we should leave things alone. We should let homoeopathy flourish in its own right, let ayurvedic medicine flourish in its own right, let allopathic medicine have its own say. Let us respect the viewpoint of others. Let us be clear where each begins and another ends, to know the limits of each. The final thing is our own consciousness. The approach we use as healers depends how far we are advanced in our own consciousness, and this affects how we treat the patients."*

Dr Mistry explained that in allopathy there were different kinds of practitioners, and he was rather dismissive of the narrow mindedness he perceived in some. He said of practitioners: *"some were so fixed, rigid and conservative that their brains have fossilised! We have to allow them to remain like that for the rest of their lives. Life will move them on. I won't move them. Then there are a fair amount of people in the intermediate range who are becoming aware of the dangers, the side effects, the toxicity, the short falls, and the pitfalls of allopathic medicine. However, they don't know what to do, because their technical training and their mind-set has been so fixed and rigid, that anything outside cannot bridge the barriers."*

"Finally there is one thin spectrum at the extreme end, those who are more open to all the new ideas. Those people are the ones who are the pioneers. They explore oriental medicine, consciousness, Zen, and Sri Aurobindo.

Those are the doctors who are coming up. The vast spectrum of around 80% who are in the middle, are both comfortable and uncomfortable, for they don't know what to do."

"I feel that mainstream medicine has got a lot of good things, but we have over used it and misused it, and now we have iatrogenic diseases. For example there is a total loss of immunity when we give vaccines to children. This is criminal. Criminal! We have to move away from that type of thinking. That is known as linear, causative, and Cartesian thinking which guided allopathy all along."

Therapeutic Systems: Religion and Health.

I asked Dr Mistry to tell me more about the relationship between religion and health. For example, if we considered religion as part of the equation, how would this benefit health? *"If understood properly, religion will help integrate the person. But with religion, like anything else, one can get stuck in the grooves. These may be grooves of ritualism, our own mindset, belief in the superiority of one religion over another, or conflicts. In those cases we loose the core teaching. Then life has to break the moulds, and people who are in those moulds suffer to a great extent."*

"Religion comes about because the core teaching becomes covered by layers of mind, which make it into dogma, into an organisation. Then once an organisation is established, it is finished: if religion becomes too one-sided, nothing much can be done."

I wondered how the ashram where I had met him in Pondicherry, of Sri Aurobindo and the Mother, fitted in with his understanding of religion. He told me *"Mother and Sri Aurobindo said they did not want their teachings to become another religion but the danger is ever present. It depends on people who follow. If you say Sri Aurobindo's yoga is the best, it is meant for all, or it is exclusive, then you have already made a religion out of it."*

"The problem is not the following of rituals, but it is the thinking process of the mind which creates the rituals. Rituals if they are done properly, in Hindu or Buddhist religions, take you towards your divinity. You will be taken towards your divinity whatever you worship. That is OK. Then there are some rituals we do blindly, not understanding what is happening. There has to come a time when the need for outer rituals will be transcended, and then you do internal rituals. At that stage the separation between 'I' and my divinity; doesn't remain."

He explained slowly, if people concentrated on the Mother, although he said that was a ritual, it would draw down the energy she could access. *"If you focus on the Mother, she was not an ordinary person. She was the holder of forces of energy and consciousness. The moment you link yourself to her, some sort of bridge occurs. That is possible in this place."*

"When I leave, I can sense a lack of this particular force, and then I have to create it in my own room, wherever I am, to make the link, an energy link. I know my guardian angels saved me from many things. If they were not looking after me, I would have been seriously injured or dead. So they kept me for religious purposes. Now I question them and challenge them."

Dr Mistry had given me so much to consider. That evening after the interview, I tried to digest his comments about the relationship between allopathic medicine, homoeopathy, religion and spirituality. His overview of the different healing modalities and the ways they could be used seemed so clear. The healing strategies were different: one tackled physicals illness, a second focused on subtle energy, and another addressed spiritual and emotional triggers. His annoyance with rigid 'fossilised' thinking of his former medical colleagues was apparent. He even questioned narrow minded religious dogma.

Medical Herbalist:
Plants and Healing

The following week, I visited Dr Loganathan, a botanist in his 30's, with a young family. He was an eye specialist, who came from a family of medical herbalists. He trained in traditional folk plant remedies, since he wanted to act as a bridge between different healing modalities. I interviewed him in his home, just outside Pondicherry. He had written a book correlating the plants with the planets and the elements. He explained about various treatments for mental ill health.

Loganathan told me his story, and explained how his forefathers, who specialised in mental health, understood the influences of planetary positions and past lives on mental health. They knew which trees should be worshipped or simply sat next to for benefit, and the plant remedies selected by a practitioner depended under what planet a person was born, and under what star. Certain plants came under the influence of certain planets. Plants could neutralise the effects of the planets on a person's mind. He gave me an example of *Calotropis*, from which the plant fibres were used to alleviate negative vibrations. It also protected children from mental illness. Using the stem fibres it could be woven as a thread around a child's waist, or made into a lamp wick, and then burned at a shrine in order to achieve mental peace and clear health. Another herb suggested for people with schizophrenia was *rawolfia serpintina*.

Loganathan completed his Masters in 1994, and then did his PhD on treatment of eye disorders, using medicinal plants. *"I was mostly working with traditional physicians when dealing with eye diseases and treating them with medicinal plants. I completed the research and my PhD in 1999, and have been practising traditional medicine systems for the last seven years, based on my hereditary experience." "In this generation, a lot of hospitals have emerged with modern facilities. There are very few traditional practitioners in this generation. Only my father is working and another elderly practitioner who treats eye diseases. Only two people are offering treatments, and their children have moved away, most do not follow the tradition."*

Since 1756, his forefathers had lived in the village of Olagapuram near Pondicherry. His ancestors had traditionally moved from one village to another, running mobile clinics in Tamil Nadu. Later the rulers of Arkot told his ancestors to settle in that village, near a well-forested area, from which they could harvest plants. The kings gave land and wanted the traditional herbalists to provide health care for people in the surrounding area. There used to be four large families, each healing different categories of disease. One specialised in eye diseases, another concentrated on bone setting, a third on child health care, including preventative health care and mental illness. The fourth family practised treatments based on astrology and horoscopes, and used chants and mantras. *"If a patient went to the wrong practitioner, he would be advised to go to the correct person, so that they would take care of him."*

Dr Loganathan's family had lived in the environs of Pondicherry for hundreds of years. He told me about his grandfather who used herbal remedies for mental heath patients. "He *looked at the individual patient's problem. He knew it is also important to consider land in their area and their horoscope. From reading the patient's horoscope one can find out the causes of their problems. Then the plants needed can be worked out for the treatment. There is no general remedy that one can give to all patients. There is one tree that practitioners advise patients to go and worship, or to sit under it in the morning or evening."* "*Plants like the nim tree, belgaum or bel tree, bilwa are also worshiped as well as kupta aromatica. This is generally good for mental health patients, but one cannot guarantee that by worshipping these plants, it will cure the illness, but it will control or suppress the problems, and the degree of the problems."*

Herbal Knowledge gained via Empathy?

I asked Loganathan how the first person ever discovered the healing qualities of plants. I wanted to know how practitioners retrieved information from plants. How did they test it, and was their knowledge achieved through occult or mechanical means? He replied: *"There are always different beliefs and reports about how the knowledge developed and was collected into book form. Saint Heztzia wrote a grammar of the Tamil language, and went into the forest and talked to the plants, to understand their qualities and actions. He did this 3 to 4000 years ago. It was more like sensing the plant".*

"When it comes to the different illnesses my father would go into the forest. He did not know the plant's name, however in those situations he just squeezed a few leaves, to smell and taste a bit, to observe the taste, and what was responsible for the smell. Then with this calculation he could say that this was good for this particular illness."

"It was more like sensing. It was like understanding the plants. We have to go into the same wavelength as the plants. The plants come to some wavelength where we can both communicate together to interrelate. It was like that."

Loganathan talked about the local sacred groves with plants where certain trees were responsible for that area's spiritual energy. *"There were sacred groves where trees were worshiped for specific reasons, and the symbol of the tree like a leaf or stem is responsible for the spiritual energy in that area. The image there and its relationship with the tree and with the land is enormous. We need to understand deeply why it is there, and how it is important for families and the whole village, or for many villages".*

Therapeutics: same symptoms, different treatment. Loganathan explained how two people with the same symptoms might require quite different treatments. Astrologically a practitioner would determine which day, week, or month each individual patient had to begin the treatment, and how long they should continue it. He told me why certain plants were needed and why their medicine needed to be worked out in each individual case.

He was interested in the supernatural aspect of plants, and their relationship with the planets and cosmos. *"I have produced this book of the plants, which are used with 27 stars, along with their botanical identity: plants used for worshipping, and a medical system for the nine planets, of worshipping plants, the reflecting areas and the influencing areas. It also says which plants are used for treatments for disease, governed by specific planets. This is correlated with the constellation and with the elements of earth, air, fire and water. The aim is to reduce problems due to an aggravation of the elements (butas) and also note the plants used by the siddhars, the ancient physicians who developed the ancient medical system. The plants used for the eight basic regulations of the human being (ashtar karma) are described in Tamil, but not yet in English".*

Grandfather's Practices. I wondered how in the past people with mental distress knew to consult with Loganathan's family members. If someone was sick, I wanted to understand how his grandfather would effect healing for mental health. He explained his grandfather would look into the horoscope of the patient, to see if he could diagnose whether it was due to a disturbance in their horoscope, or to another person's horoscope. *"In some horoscopes we can see that the father and his son should not be resident in the same place. After ten years if there has been a separation, then both can become well. From there we can ask the question, what is the situation in your family?"*

"First we look to see if the problem is due to some family members, and if it is not due to that, it may be due to some planet. What is suited to the patient is worked out, and if it is due to planetary inferences, they will be advised to go to different temples for the relevant planet. For example if a marriage is being delayed due to the influence of the planet, the patient

is advised to go to the relevant planet temple situated in different parts of the country."

"There is one literature called yoga sutra, which gives all the problems for mental illness, which may be due to hereditary effects. That means the different karmas, and the different actions performed, not by the patient, but the patient's father or forefathers. That leads to this problem in this generation. That means the ending of the karma, the ending of that evil action. It stops there, so that the next generation of that family will be normal."

Therapeutics: Plants and Planets.

What other combinations of factors did his grandfather consider for conditions like hysteria or depression? What treatment options were there? His response was more complex than my question: *"It is not so generalised. It is not so easy, because the causes of mental health are due to different factors. For example mental illness in the village region is entirely different from mental patients in the city areas. Even the causes are not related. When it occurs in the city areas, it is due to drug abuse, alcohol abuse, financial reasons, and family separations. These are the main problems we see when patients from the towns. When patients come from the villages it is mainly social problems."*

I asked Loganathan to explain more about specific plants for treatments, which were given at astrologically correct times. *"Using calculations based on a patient's birth chart, one can determine the good and bad times of the patient. But also going in deep to calculate the degrees of the elevation of the planet, and linking that with their lifetime, one can note that this time, this particular planet has a major role influencing this person. We can determine the peak period of this planet on this person, and the peak period for the plant's healing."*

"There are planets responsible for health and education, and family. Each planet has different responsibilities, according to its combination

with others. One has to see the degree of elevation of each planet to see whether they cause mental illness. Alternatively mental ill health could be due to other members of the family, which must be taken into consideration.

"If we don't look at all of this, we may misunderstand the horoscope, and then the plant selected for treatment may not be the most helpful."

Loganathan mentioned certain plants were correlated to certain planets, and this influenced their relationship for treatment systems. *"Once you have worked out the real cause of mental health, then we can look at what plant can be used to alleviate the effect of this planet. For example in the case of the moon, which plays a major role in determining the mind of a human being, one plant called bute monstera plays a major role in the worshipping of planet moon. So worshipping this plant and giving medicine from it would lead to a reduction of the symptoms. There is another one called plumeria alba which can be worshipped, and flowers can be taken which lead to a reduction of mental symptoms."*

He told me about the Bio-resource Centre, established at Pitchandikulam in Auroville, for the protection and propagation of medicinal plants. This was one of a network of Medicinal Plant Conservation Parks in south India. The focus of this forest sanctuary was on conserving and documenting indigenous plants with medicinal properties. They collected and propagated seeds in their nursery, and created a living gene bank of plant species. They supplied medical herbal practitioners with herbs and seedlings, and arranged support meetings for information sharing. They empowered villagers to care for the forest, which provided them with resources, and thus they encouraged the continuity of ancient cultural traditions. I thanked Loganathan for so much depth of information and returned to Pondicherry.

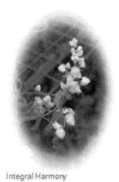

Integral Harmony

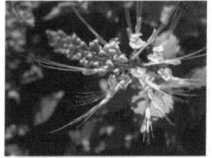

Spiritual Intensity, photo by Mr Sircar

❖ ❖ ❖

The American Psychiatrist:
Allopathy and Flower Remedies

The following week, I sat on the low circular wall just outside the Ashram Dining Halls. The lunch period was over, and people were streaming out of the halls, chatting to each other. As the crowds thinned out, I began to chat quietly with Dr Michael Miovic[41], [42]. An American psychiatrist, he worked at the Dana Farber Cancer Institute, Boston, and was a colleague of Dr Basu. He held deep understanding of psychology: its profound aspects and the way psychology, psychiatry and soul healing worked together.

He worked in Harvard in an oncology ward of a hospital, and suggested his patients use flower remedies to enhance their psychological well being. I told him I'd been prescribed some flower remedies myself, one called Integral Harmony, to help me get in touch with my soul's purpose, and hopefully ease underlying depression. I was told it was a creeper, with a small white bell shaped flower, which died suddenly and then regenerated.

At the time of our conversation, Dr Miovic was completing a fellowship in psychosocial oncology. He frequently visited Pondicherry, as he had aligned himself to the philosophy of the sage Sri Aurobindo. He explained how he used remedies with USA patients: *"I use flower remedies primarily with outpatients who are dealing with depression, anxiety, low self-esteem, and/or traumatic memories. I have not yet used flower remedies with people who are in the middle of psychotic or manic states, because those conditions are more severe and therefore there are both scientific and medico-legal reasons to use more established treatments for them. In the United States, one has more latitude to negotiate the use of complementary/alternative methods of treatment with mid-to high-functioning patients than with those with severe mental illness."*

I wondered how he presented the remedies in that hospital, and what effect they had with patients who had cancer. He explained: *"Because cancer is life threatening and there are often no scientifically validated cures, patients may pursue every kind of alternative treatment available. The advantage of using Bach flower essences, again, is that they are safe to combine with chemotherapy and radiation treatment, and there are some standard formulations (such as Rescue Remedy and Rock Rose) that are useful for fear, panic, and mental/physical trauma, feelings that are rife in cancer treatment".*

"Obviously, both medical and surgical treatments for cancer can be traumatic in many ways, as they are psychologically and physically invasive, and patients are often emotionally paralysed by the fear of death. Sometimes this fear is appropriate, for the situation really is grim, while other times it is in excess of the medical and surgical severity of the situation. But in either case, fear is fear and it has a tremendous psychological impact on the patient, so I find flower essences quite helpful here."

Flower Remedies, Soul and Psychology. I asked Dr Miovic to explain to me the connection between flowers and our soul, and between psychiatry and the soul. I hadn't realised his (and The Mother's) explicit connection between human soul and the healing effect of flowers. He said: *"Mother says that flowers express the soul consciousness only through silence and beauty. But they don't have language, they can't speak, they don't have any mental body, so they cannot express consciousness in the same mental form like us."*

"The flower essences are a unique opportunity to bring a psychic vibration into psychotherapy and the treatment of emotional issues. The 'vital' in Sri Aurobindo's system is where emotions occur. But there is a possibility for a potentially even higher form."

He continued: *"If we are actually conscious of our soul and psychic being, and so in tune with it that we can manifest it in action and work, then we could also do psychotherapy and make interpretations that are language and mental expressions, that carry direct psychic intuition and insight, and express it in language. So there is the possibility within psychotherapy of developing a truly psychic (from the soul) psychotherapy, but it takes a lot of discipline and learning."*

I asked Dr Miovic about the relationship between western transpersonal psychology and soul medicine. He explained: *"Transpersonal could mean anything non-material, or anything that is not studied in classic ego psychology. It is a vast realm. For instance transpersonal could be 'prana' or acupuncture and herbs. If you accept the fact that 'chi' exists, that is transpersonal, but it is not the soul. You could go up into other occult areas such as astrology and astral realms: these are transpersonal but not the soul."*

"Sri Aurobindo describes ranges of mental opening and intuition of the human mind, the higher mind, and the over mind. It is transpersonal but it is not the soul. The realm of what is transpersonal is vast."

"*Sri Aurobindo and Mother are very specific. When they say soul, they mean the psychic being, which is something very specific. It is an important distinction which transpersonal psychology does not always understand.*"

I asked whether the term 'psychic being' pertained to human beings rather than anything else, and wanted to know exactly what Sri Aurobindo and the Mother meant by this. "*Their idea is that the psychic is the nucleus of the divine consciousness that evolves in the world. The psychic is present in plants and animals but it is informed, like an atmosphere that coalesces and dissolves. So when they mean the psychic being, they mean the actual soul, that incarnation from life to life which follows an evolutionary path, from unorganised matter all the way up to the highest spiritual saints and sages and beyond.*"

He continued: "*when we die our bodies will dissolve: the prana goes, the subtle physical dissolves, the inner vital being and mental being dissolve. Only some inner essence of anything you have learnt in your life remains, but not the full formation.*"

He informed me about his understanding of rebirth: "*when you are reborn, you have a capacity. If you had an intense development in music in a past life, you'll have an appreciation of music in this life, but it doesn't mean that you can play every single piece you used to know how to play. There are certain levels of reality, which dissolve upon death. So when they say psychic beings, Mother means specifically that. She says the flowers actually express that essential concept.*"

I questioned whether this meant that when a practitioner used flower remedies, he or she was treating like with like. I was curious to know about the healing modality, how these remedies compared with homoeopathy. "*Yes, like with like, and that is an interesting difference between bio-medicine and homoeopathy, and it was the reason that Bach developed the flower remedies. He was a homoeopath* and he said 'why are we giving someone a toxin, when you shake it and percuss it to capture its vibration, you are concentrating and purifying a negative vibration, and then you use it as a vaccine. You introduce that negative vibration into your subtle physical atmosphere and you develop a tolerance for it, react against it, and overcome it. It is just like in the physical level, using physical vaccines. They are effective."

"But he was interested in why people had to use negative vibrations and he asked himself why not use something purely positive. So that is what led him to this intuition that the most positive things he could find were flowers. So he concentrated on that vibration, to introduce that vibration into the healing system."

Flower remedies and mental well being. I asked Dr Miovic about Integral Yoga, and how it influenced psychological well being, the 'vital' and the emotional body (terms I had heard used in the ashram: 'vital' meant a force which governed emotions). He described what he understood about integral health and psychotherapy: "Integral yoga brings a higher force to that path, so I am interested in a synthesis of those two. Psychotherapy over the last hundred years has come to a broad consensus among many different schools of psychology. There is a defensive process: the vital, when it feels pain, whether it is fear or grief or sadness or an excitation that is taboo, or is not allowed, or painful to experience, it protects itself and hides that from the ego's awareness."

He advised me flower remedies performed by healing deep psychological issues. I inquired exactly what was favourable about using flower essences, and I asked him how they related to a person's psychological state. "Flower therapies are great because at best they are helpful additions to the range of modalities I may use, while at worst they are placebos. They have no drug-drug interactions, and side effects are practically nil. This is quite different from herbal medicines, which are pharmacologically active and therefore have a greater range of potential side effects and drug-herb interactions."

"Flower essences are also particularly useful for psychotherapy because they are prescribed according to psychological states and personality profiles that are very familiar to therapists and psychiatrists.... You hear so much intimate material from your clients that it is not difficult to identify their salient emotional problems and personality style."

Dr Miovic pointed out how he thought remedies worked on human beings, although he was aware little research had yet been done on efficacy. *"I believe that flower essences have real effects on the mental and vital bodies. Of course, this is only a personal belief as yet, since I do not have brain scans or even the results of simple clinical trials to prove an actual treatment effect. However, that data may emerge in the future, and even if it doesn't, flower essences will remain good placebos at worst, and at best may be thought of as energy-treatments that work in unquantifiable ways."*

Flower remedies were used by some members of the ashram's medical team to provide healing for patients at the Beach Office in Pondicherry. I was interested in exploring further ways practitioners used them, and I wanted to know more about the different healing modalities the various remedies used. I asked Dr Miovic to clarify this, and I summarise his comments below.

Dr Miovic's Healing Modalities of Remedies

The psychiatrist Dr Michael Miovic explained the following concepts to raise awareness of different ways each remedy worked:
- Allopathic medicine uses pharmacologically active ingredients
- Herbal remedies use natural pharmacology, and are pharmacologically active
- *Acupuncture works on energy flows, chi or pranic energy, which is more vital or vital-physical*
- Homoeopathy treats like with like and affects the subtle physical body. Homoeopathy treats the whole person, not the parts. The patient is given a homoeopathic dose of a

toxin, which induces the same symptoms as the illness. *"Then the body's subtle physical and vital sheaths react against this low dose toxic vibration, and learn to overcome it"*

- Flower remedies: Dr Bach wondered why people used negative or toxic vibrations, and decided to try positive energy instead. He intuited *"flowers are the most positive and spiritually nourishing life form in the mineral and vegetable kingdoms."* He experimented with making homoeopathic preparations of flowers, treating a condition with its antidote or opposition.

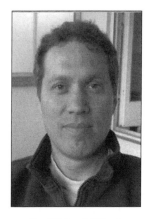

Dr Michael Miovic

Dr Miovic explained differences between healing modalities of alternative therapies, which are set out above. From the perspective of Integral Yoga, he said flower essences were the first medical treatment modality that worked at the level of psychic consciousness. He stressed they evoked the vibrational level of the true soul. The Mother was aware that of the entire vegetable kingdom, flowers alone expressed the vibration of the psychic (i.e. true soul) worlds.

I hadn't realised explicitly, that there was a vibrational connection between flowers and the soul, and between psychiatry and the soul. Dr Miovic continued: *"Mother says flowers express the soul consciousness only through silence and beauty, as they can't speak and have no mental body. Thus, flowers cannot express the psychic consciousness as fully as a spiritually developed human being. However, since the average person is too preoccupied with their mental and vital activities to be clearly aware of the psychic being, flowers can serve as a useful way of reminding us to connect with this psychic feeling and psychic consciousness. This affords us new avenues for psychotherapeutic treatment."*

"I should also point out that there also exists a possibility for developing an even higher form of therapy than flower remedies. If human beings can become fully conscious of our soul (psychic being), and so in tune with it that we can manifest it in action and work, then we could also do psychotherapy and make interpretations that carry direct psychic intuition and insight."

"Bach had the correct intuition that flowers are the most positive and spiritually nourishing life form in the mineral and vegetable kingdoms, and so he experimented with making homeopathic preparations of flowers. As a result, in flower therapy you are actually treating by antidote or by opposition: if the person is fearful, you give a flower that has the positive vibration of courage; if they are grief-stricken, you give one that fills the heart with sweetness."

I was curious as to how Dr Miovic, a conventional psychiatrist would present the healing properties of flower remedies to his own patients in the USA. He explains: *"I tell patients that flower remedies are related to homeopathy. That is, they are herbal preparations that are entirely non-pharmacological. If the person seems open-minded or expresses interest in spirituality or complementary/ alternative medicine, I will also say that flower essences are a type of energetic medicine. And if they are really open or love flowers, I will speak a little bit about the unique beauty and vibrational consciousness of flowers, and perhaps weave in a few comments about the soul and spirituality."*

"However, if the person is not so open to these things, I will simply present flower remedies as an absolutely safe, non-addictive, non-pharmacological alternative that may be of some help, but certainly cannot hurt. If they ask about scientific studies, I say that there are some studies that suggest homeopathy can be helpful for certain conditions, but as yet few case-studies involving flower remedies. I then re-emphasize the fact that, at worst, flower remedies will have no effect, either positive or negative. In the United States, because of frequent

medical lawsuits, I ask patients to buy their own Bach remedies at the health-food store."

"I am hopeful that scientific studies will be done on flower essences in the future. I think that a functional MRI study of people taking flower essences would be fascinating, and if a positive result were found, that would really challenge the current biochemical model of consciousness. For if a flower essence is just a placebo, how can it alter mood and feeling in a specific way that plain water does not, unless there is indeed some sort of subtle energy that mediates the effect?"

SUMMARY

I was overwhelmed by information generated by the levels of awareness of each professional practitioner I interviewed. That is, their spiritual awareness of therapeutic strategies and healing modalities went profoundly beyond my own. I felt I was not in a position to evaluate or judge their knowledge: my aim was simply to present the recorded interview data with as much clarity as possible.

I received new insight into flower remedies and the ways they were used to intervene in matters of the soul and psychology. I had learnt about the significance of flowers in terms of the Mother's philosophy. The explanations comparing the healing modalities between flower remedies, homoeopathy, herbal medicine, and allopathy was very illuminating.

The interview with the medical herbalist, who came from a long family tradition of practitioners, brought up information about the relationship of herbalism to astrology, and the correlation of planetary systems with states of mental ill health. He described the way the original herbalists empathetically acquired knowledge about plants. The interview data presented informants' own beliefs about their work. Whether we claim this material is 'belief' or 'knowledge' depends on our judgement of our own frameworks of understanding.

The interview with the homoeopathic physician illustrated ways homoeopathy had been used in collaboration with allopathic doctors. I was most interested in the surgeon who had turned to homoeopathy, and questioned what he perceived to be the rigid thinking of allopathic doctors, his former colleagues, and rigid rituals of some religions. In contrast I heard about the psychiatrist who practiced western models of psychiatry with low maintenance dose western pharmacology, but also suggested his patients engage in supportive religious rituals and practices.

In the following chapter I continue on the theme of treatment strategies, and present results of fieldwork trips to address syncretic religious and spiritual practices for the treatment of mental well being. I explore worship, pilgrimage and healing rituals in specific places in South India. I start by presenting places renowned for healing mental distress, and then in the following chapter, I set out places which pilgrims visit for mental peace.

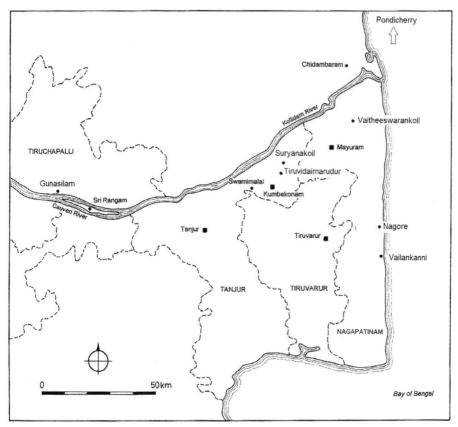

Figure 3   Tanjur and surrounding districts

Chapter Six

RELIGIOUS ESTABLISHMENTS FOR MENTAL DISTRESS

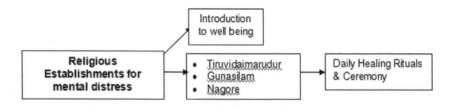

Introduction: Religious Activities for well being

Alongside pharmacological treatments and therapeutic remedies, patients sought relief from their mental distress by visiting Hindu temples, Christian churches, or Muslim shrines. I visited three religious establishments in Tamil Nadu renowned for addressing mental distress: Tiruvidaimarudur, Gunasilam, and Nagore.

People not only travelled to religious places appropriate to their faith of birth, but also undertook pilgrimages to healers and priests in places of different religions. They used amulets appropriate to whatever religious place they had approached, which would be worn around the waist, shoulders, upper arms, wrists or neck. Patients undertook rituals with healers, whatever the religion, and allowed prayers to be said over them. Sometimes they felt there was more 'power' for healing with a religious practitioner of another faith.

This chapter explores religious and spiritual treatment strategies for healing mental distress and mental peace. I discovered that the term 'mental health' was a western usage, and people I spoke to in Calcutta and Tamil Nadu were not familiar with it, so I have used mental distress and mental peace throughout.

During the fieldwork years, I visited two ashrams, five temples, a cathedral and a mosque in the Tamil Nadu area, and observed or participated in rituals in each one. Dr Basu asked two of his Tamil-speaking colleagues to accompany me on tours around temples, and I am very grateful to each of them. In rural areas, where there were less available government health care facilities for the mentally distressed, it was the custom to send patients to holy places to receive the vibrations of the deities or saints, in order to cure them of their afflictions.

The use of temples, churches and mosques for alleviating mental distress is covered in depth here, together with rituals devotees and pilgrims engaged in. I travelled around several sites in Tamil Nadu, visiting places renowned to be healing for those with mental distress, and stayed in the town of Vaitheeswaraakoil, famous for its palm leaf oracle libraries.

Prayer or direct contact with the divine or with realised beings was said to enhance mental well-being. This was achieved through prayer and mediation at ashrams such as those of Sri

Aurobindo and SriRamana Maharshi. Each ashram offered residential accommodation for devotees. Direct access was said to cut through all the outer layers of spiritual existence and the layers where disembodied beings co-exist and interact with humans. These ashrams were not considered appropriate places for those with mental disorders because the '*force was so great*'.

Those people who were mid to high functioning or with chronic conditions participated in religious rituals to enhance their mental well-being. They propitiated deities on specific days of the week, and paid their respects to deified images of the nine the planets, which were found at most south Indian temples. They offered prayers and undertook devotion in front of the shrines of Hindu deities. They chanted mantras and offered sacrifices of vegetable (coconuts) or living creatures (hens), or fire (camphor) and smoke (incense). I was told: "*People received mantras from a guru, as part of their initiation package. When they said the mantra, they tuned into the energy of all the repeated mantras, and this energised their requests and activities.*" Pilgrims made a tour of different temples: they hung prayers on sacred trees within temple compounds as at Tiruvidaimarudur. They walked up sacred hills such as Arunchalai at Tiruvanamalai, or bathed in sacred water tanks in Vaitheeswarankoil.

At Suryanakoil pilgrims visited the temple to propitiate planets that influenced their health. At Vaitheeswarankoil they commissioned priests to perform prayer rituals on their behalf. In the temple at Rameshwaram, they performed ablutions at the 22 wells for their mental well-being, and conducted water-side prayers for their deceased relatives. At Gunasilam, where the temple was renowned for its healing properties, people travelled long distances (up to 6 hours) on Sunday to take part in the anointing ceremonies at the inner shrine. Men and women alike would wear amulets and charms, some made of silver with tiny scrolls of prayer rolled or folded inside.

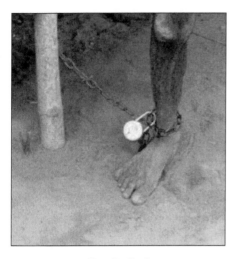

Foot Padlock

People with acute mental illness engaged in all of the above, but before the government ban in the year 2000, some were taken to temples and mosques and restrained there. Chained in the vicinity of the shrine, they bathed in the vibrations of the deity or saint, and this was believed to heal their mental disorders. After the government ban, people were still taken to these places, but they could only remain there if a relative stayed with them and guided them through the rituals. For example the mosque at Nagore had thick rings embedded into columns where the mentally ill had been chained. None were in use during my visit, although relatives attended some sick people who were there. Attendants performed cleansing rituals at the tombs of the saints, and these were intended to remove any impurities or disembodied spirits from the person.

At the first temple visited, I met carers at an asylum and several men held chained within a hut outside the compound walls. However, after this visit chaining stopped. There had been a fire at Muslim shrine in Chennai, where many mentally ill people had been held. Thirty men chained there had died in the fire, so the State decreed no more people should be chained, and asked for them all to be sent home to their relatives.

Since that time all the men in the hut outside had gone. A newspaper cutting from 5th February 2002, said the Supreme

Court had directed each of the States must *"ensure that none of the patients in any of the mental asylums in the country be chained."* That it should be the responsibility of each area's police station *"to ensure the closure of an unlicensed mental asylum and shift the patients to a nearby government mental hospital"*. After the government ban on restraint, when I revisited holy places where people with mental distress were taken for healing, the only patients seen were accompanied. The visit described below took place before the ban.

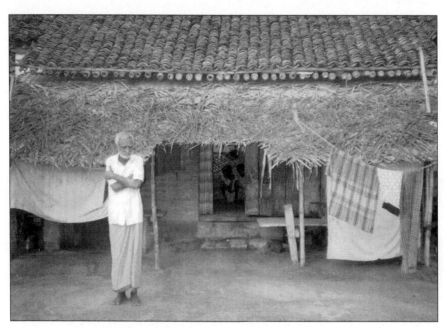

Asylum at South gate of the Mahalingam temple, with carer

Tiruvidaimarudur: Mahalingam temple

In Pondicherry, the driver picked me up at the hotel at 3.30am and Dr Pani (one of Dr Basu's colleagues, an ophthalmologist whose hobby was temple photography and who spoke Tamil) and I travelled through the night driving through scenery of beautiful shades of grey; flat paddy fields, palm trees reflected in water, and a clear sky with lots of stars. I experienced such a sense of peace, within the soft grey sky and mysterious grey lands, driving slowly past a winding river with houses built right on its banks. There were so few cars or bikes that the inhabitants used the road to sleep on. I felt calm, at peace, and extremely tired, for I'd hardly had any sleep. The roads were very quiet and rather dark. A white Mercedes drove past us at speed. Half an hour later, we drove past it: having taken a sharp corner at speed, it ended up in the bushes. The driver and passengers stood beside it. Later on the journey I was excited to see five buzzards, a hawk with a white belly, and a huge flock of cranes.

We were driving to the home of Naganathan, head priest from the Sri Murugan Temple in London. His parents lived near Mayuram, and he was in India due to tragic circumstances. His young wife had died some weeks earlier, on a hospital operating table in London. She was only 35, and he had brought her body back to its final resting place in India, together with his two daughters and young son.

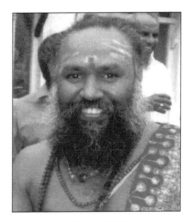

Naganathan, Sri Murugan Temple, London

Although the day we met him was one of ceremony to support his wife's spirit and the family's wellbeing, he drove out with us to introduce us to some priests, accompanied by many of his family. The date was very auspicious. Once in every 150 years certain planets came into alignment, and we visited a temple in Mayuram for special prayers. I was so grateful he accompanied us on that day.

We drove to the temple at Tiruvidaimarudur, renowned for housing the mentally disturbed, past tiny roads, wrecked by the recent hurricane. There were many trees down, and monkeys on the road were investigating the fallen trees. At the temple we were dropped at the north entrance while Naganathan a Brahmin priest was dropped at the west entrance.

Outside the south gate was a row of simple houses, in which the mentally disturbed were chained. Those with epilepsy and severe learning difficulties were excluded. Eight men who seemed subdued and calm, were chained by the ankle. There were two men on each bench and others inside. From within another man peered out, with just his head and hand visible, his body hidden behind the door: he wanted to talk with the charismatic Naganathan.

I learnt later that the hut was an economic enterprise: it had nothing to do with the temple or the priests, who played no part in the care of the mentally distressed, other than performing their regular prayer rituals. This was a commercial operation, from which the owners got money from relatives, and it did not necessarily benefit the men themselves, who came from various parts of Tamil Nadu (chart 6.1). People heard of the asylum by word of mouth: others spoke about the temple and its cures.

CHART NO.6.1 JANUARY 2001: MEN STAYING IN HUT BY TIRUVIDAIMARUDUR TEMPLE			
Name	native place	caste	length of stay
Male T.N.K	Tiruvidaimarudur		
Male M.R	Kumbakonam	chettiar	
Male R.J	Pattikottai	naidu	3-4 months
Male H	Madras	kallar	7-8 months
Male A.P	Myladutherai	ayyar, Brahmin	12 months
Male B	Nagapattinam	Telugu chettiar	6 months
Male R	Rameshwaram	chettiar	6 months
Male Vi	Mallipattinam-Pudukottai	fisherman	30 days
Male Ve	*Pudukottai*	*ayyar, Brahmin*	*20 days*

Daily Ritual. The men in chains were woken up around 7.00 am in the cold days of winter. They slept and ate inside the hut, and they were manacled at night. One, who talked to himself all the time and appeared to be very angry, was chained at the wrist, whereas all the others were manacled on the ankle. One frail-looking elderly man, who spoke good English, said he had been there for 28 years, first as an inmate and now free. He helped out as a carer for the others.

After waking, the men were escorted by their carers, and walked south down the road to a wide natural lake where they all bathed. One carer was a well-educated young man in his 20's: the Naidu owner's son, responsible for the men in the hut. His family provided food for the men. After bathing the men then filed back into the temple by the south gate and started their tour of the shrines. They paid homage to the main deity Mahalingam, and went to each shrine making a complete circuit around the whole complex.

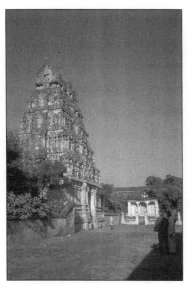

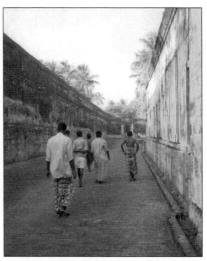

*Temple walkway during
perambulation*

*Temple walkways used by
the mentally distressed at
Tiruvidaimarudur*

Carer's story. One man walked over to us. Karun was a priest's attendant, wearing a white cloth lunghi, and carrying papers in a plastic bag. A thin man with a gaunt face, haunting black eyes, long straggling black hair, he had vowed a life of celibacy. A native of Tiruvidaimarudur itself, he assisted priests in the inner sanctum of the temple as they performed prayer rituals, and helped the poor.

He explained the men had been brought from outside villages, by their relatives who paid three or four caretakers to look after them, and cook their food. Once in the morning and once in the afternoon they were unchained and escorted into the temple through the south gate. They walked around the precincts, from south to west, north to east. They did this for a 'mangalam', a period of 48 or 60 days, after which many of them were believed cured.

While we were talking with him, another man came up. He was a sanyasi (a begging monk) formerly from Madurai. A talkative stocky man in his 60's, with long white hair and a beard, he had excellent English. He said he used to be an accountant with a large company, but had given up everything for the life of a wandering monk, living simply in white robes, and begging for his food.

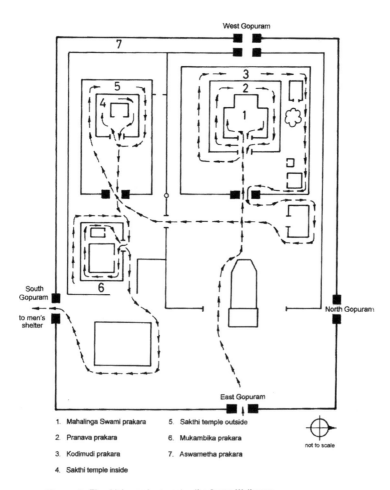

Figure 4 Tiruvidaimarudur temple: the Seven Walkways

1. Mahalinga Swami prakara
2. Pranava prakara
3. Kodimudi prakara
4. Sakthi temple inside
5. Sakthi temple outside
6. Mukambika prakara
7. Aswametha prakara

Healing place and perambulation. Both men walked with us, for one entire length of the outer precinct, starting from south to north. They explained how a cure for mental distress occurred during the perambulation. Karun said the place was very healing, and it changed the men's vibration. Along the walkway, many sacred herbs grew freely, and our companions said these also helped change the energy of mentally disturbed people. There was a line along the path and the men walked one-side of it or the other. We were told underneath the ground, at unknown places, sacred artefacts of a holy person were buried, which caused healing vibrations to radiate upwards. There were so many healing factors connected with this temple.

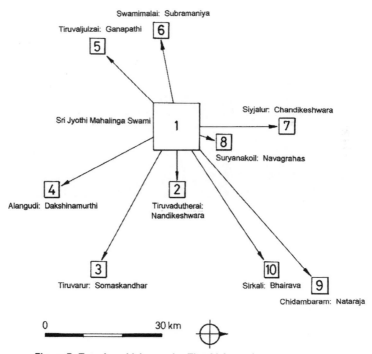

Figure 5 Temples which energise Tiruvidaimarudur

According to paintings along one wall in the inner corridors, this temple was at the central point of nine other temples on a 50 mile radius. It had a huge ShivaLingam, known as Mahalingam. It was at the centre point of four Shiva temples, and received energy from all of them (figure 4 above). All this energy went towards the healing of mentally disturbed people.

A story about the temple being beneficial for healing mental distress was told in paintings around the walls: by accident, a king on horseback killed a brahmin, whose spirit cursed and chased him. The king hid in the temple in distress: as the spirit could not come in. The king found walking around the shrines made him feel better mentally, and was freed of his mental disturbance.

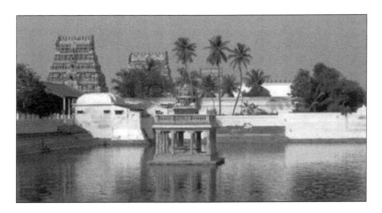

Temple tank at Tiruvidaimarudur

Dr Basu had visited rural asylums with us, and seen the circumstances of the inpatients. Even though unsupervised restraint was no longer appropriate in India, he considered the sacred rituals may indeed be of benefit to the inmates. He made suggested for their upkeep, and thought the following modifications could be made to the service for patients:

- Patients should be offered more adequate living accommodation, and they should not be chained, but should be medicated if necessary.
- A more regular treatment strategy should be created, which incorporated temple rituals, healing rituals and other healing therapies.
- That the rituals around the temple should continue, supplemented by medication
- That the manager should be invited to co-operate, to build a mental health institute, to keep the spirit of care intact, but change the outer forms in accordance with the times.
- Specialists well versed in the occult, should come to the temple to determine its significance.
- A plan would be developed for a sacred architecture project, relevant to that site, that was in consonance with the temple, and conducive to the patient's welfare.

He thought the above combination would be most appropriate for these patients, so as well as the religious walking, they should also be treated in a better environment. He suggested the men at Tiruvidaimarudur should continue to go around the temple but their regime should be supplemented by medicine.

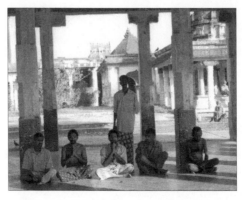

Men with their carer sitting outside a shrine

Discussions about the future

One afternoon, a few of us convened at Dr Basu house. We met to discuss the possibility of constructing a purpose built asylum on a parcel of land near the temple. I learnt The Mother in one of her notes on Auroville envisioned there would be a new healing centre for the sick, developed using a consciousness based and spiritually appropriate architecture.

We had earlier discussed the development of an asylum to house the mentally ill, so they would live in better conditions, have access to modern medication, and still perform temple rituals. Since that time Dr Basu had spoken to the head priest, who was willing for us to build near the temple, and would give land on which to do so. Apparently the head priest mentioned a visit to the town of Vaitheeswarankoil, where he had consulted the libraries of inscribed palm leaves. The reading he received said it was written many thousand years ago, that people would come from elsewhere, to construct a building. The palm leaves mentioned the kind of land they should be offered, that it should be rectangular, of a particular size, with a stream at one edge.

Sadly as we talked, stories of corruption emerged. The senior Pontiff at the monastery, which administered 50 or 60 shrines, had already appointed his successor. According to the astrologer who read the palm leaf texts, it was written… that we should pay the successor an 'unaccounted sum of money' (that is a bribe) in order to get the right piece of land. We all agreed this was inappropriate since it would set a model of deceit from the start. The Pontiff's successor wanted us to have a much poorer piece of land, which was not the correct shape mentioned in the palm leaf oracles.

Since none of our group spoke or read Tamil, Dr Basu felt the interpreters of the palm leaf texts could say whatever they felt like. He doubted very much whether the ancient authors of these texts would have suggested a bribe. However the doctor suggested that rather than pay a bribe, we would not use temple land, and would buy a plot elsewhere to set up the Trust.

Dr Basu told us a team of mental health professionals and architects from Auroville were researching and studying the temple site in order to replicate its principles in a modern manner in Auroville. Their brief was to give consideration to aesthetic principles, and the local flora and fauna. The design should provide healing spaces which cater to different planes of consciousness in a human being. For example, one space should be appropriate to treatment using pharmacology, another to psychological therapeutic work, another to artists and musicians, and another used to focus on the body. One space would support the integration of all these aspects around higher principles. Treatment would be offered in the light of Sri Aurobindo's philosophy.

The centre at Auroville to treat and investigate psychological disorders was envisaged as residential, with therapy rooms mentioned above, acute wards, office spaces, and kitchen and dining areas. The design originally considered for the healing centre was oriented around a grid, which would provide energetic order: to merge lessons of the past with present insights to move into the future. Dr Basu explained "*at both the physical and the metaphorical centre, this space fuses the energies of the Divine from above with the energies of manifestation from below, and around this space patients can meditate upon their journeys and contemplate their return to the world outside.*"

Gunasilam Temple

The following week, we were told about another temple in Tiruchappali, where the deity specialised in supporting patients with mental distress. We hired a car and drove to Gunasilam, a small village with a Vaishnava temple, near the Cauvery River. The temple housed one shrine to Sri Prasanna Venkateshwara, who was said to be the 'happy' elder brother of Venkateshwara at Tirupathi. The deity was said to be as powerful as the one at Tirupathi, and after a visit here a pilgrim would expect to derive the same benefit. The temple was built around 1800 AD. Across the road was a small tank, with water lilies and a dainty central mandapa.

On either side of the temple were rows of houses with 'caged' verandas, which could be locked. Some were occupied and had clothes hanging. Due to the government ban on unaccompanied mental health patients, there were very few visitors here. However, pilgrims regularly came from Chennai to visit this place for prophylactic purposes, since it brought so much mental peace. On the day we arrived, one woman had travelled for six hours to reach here, and had come with eight other family members.

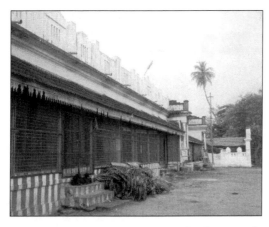

Gunasilam empty caged verandas, formally for the mentally disturbed

There was only one small cafe in the village, with seating for about eight people. Pilgrims were served off a banana leaf plate: when we had finished eating, we folded the leaf and dropped it into an outlet to the street wall, from where dogs, crows and cows could feed on them. While we sat there, two female pilgrims came in to collect food parcels. The woman in charge of this cafe also looked after the welfare of the mentally ill, and cooked their meals. There were many fewer distressed patients here due to the government response after the fire in Madras: this meant patients would only come if accompanied by their relatives.

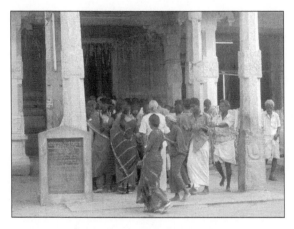

Gunasilam queue for ceremony

Anointing ceremony. At each prayer ceremony in the temple there was an anointing ritual. We queued with pilgrims and patients and once we reached the front by the shrine, we were splashed violently in the face with *tulasi* water (basil). This was quite shocking as I was not expecting it. Usually prayers were said five times a day: 6.30, 7.30, 10.30, 5.30, and 8.30. Patients were invited to chant a mantra 108 times, twice a day: this was "*om namu naraiyana*". We were told patients had to be chained, for without chains it was difficult to restrain them. There was a charge of 50 rupees a day for the temple to provide the rooms, in addition to the fee for the worshiping ceremony of '*archana*'.

We visited the place on a Sunday, when there were many visitors from outside. At 12.30 in the afternoon there was a special *abishekam*, or anointing ceremony. Around 100 people arrived in vans and cars for the ceremony in this small temple. They queued outside into the street. All were queuing to get relief from mental affliction and spirit attachment.

The mentally ill were usually first in line, guided by their relatives. They received a vigorous splashing of holy water in the face, and it shocked some. This shock was considered necessary to remove any attached discarnate spirits. When long-term patients arrived at the temple, they were given silver charms or amulets, which were worn for ten or fifteen days, in order to release them from mental ailments. The charms were made in silver and then energised by the deity, in a ceremony carried out inside the temple, with a basket of flowers and other offerings for the deity. Then the amulet could be tied to a male's right wrist and a female's left wrist. These amulets were spiritually charged so they protected the wearer for a specific length of time.

Nagore Mosque

That afternoon, we were informed Nagore mosque was considered an important site for healing mental distress, so we headed towards the Bay of Bengal coast. People of all faiths came to this mosque from near and far, believing vibrations of Muslim saints would heal them and their relatives of mental afflictions. The attendants, priests and pilgrims believed the presiding saint's energy was so powerful it drove out spirits and evil forces that attacked human beings. This was effective whether one was Muslim, Hindu or Christian. Everyone could be cured or receive mental peace. The Hindu Ayappa in their black robes and black beards passed through here as part of their pilgrimage.

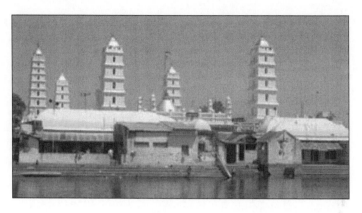

Nagore Mosque

The Mosque and its associated buildings covered a huge area, and had five minarets to represent the five main tenets of Islam. The complex housed three *samadhis:* the tomb of a great Muslim saint, Hazarath Sayed Mohamed Yousef who died at Nagore in 1570 AD (978h), and those of his wife and son.

Guide book texts. According to the guide book[43], saint Hazarath Sayed Mohamed Yousef was born in 1501 AD (909h) to parents in Manickappur in Uttar Pradesh. His father was himself descended from a mystical order of saints. As a youth he sacrificed himself to Allah, and at eighteen he left for Guwalior in Madhya Pradesh. He undertook concentrated meditation and continued to perform miracles to help the needy, sick and poor. He travelled to Mecca and Medina for six years before returning to Lahore.

Then he moved to Nagore on the Bay of Bengal, which at that time was just a few fishermen huts. There he developed astral body projection, left his body and travelled to a sacred shrine in Sri Lanka, where he left his hand imprint on the wall. After

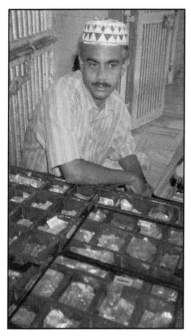

Amulet seller

refusing marriage a number of times, he eventually took a wife, Sayed Sultan Beeri Shahiba (whose tomb was next to his in the complex) and who bore him six sons and two daughters. When he left his body for the last time, his son recited obsequies above his grave, and he was heard to reply from the tomb. In 1570 a thatched roof was put over the grave. As the flow of offerings began, fishermen erected walls around the grave, and built a domed roof above. Pilgrims began to visit, as its healing properties became renowned.

Each of the three *samadhis* had an attendant at its front entrance, which opened onto a white tiled, neon-lit chamber. Pilgrims entered by side doors. They rested their head on the wall by the *samadhi*, touching the Arabic text inscribed on the surface. Some visitors suddenly made a sharp sound: said to release any afflictions they had within. One man sitting on his own kept yelling out sporadically. Prior to the government ban on shrine asylums, this had been a major place where the mentally disturbed were brought by their relatives.

Prophylactic amulets. Outside the tomb complex, but within the walls of the mosque, was a seller of silvered aluminium amulets. These amulets were mainly for people with physical problems, but some were specifically for those with mental problems. There were hundreds of eyes, legs and arms, hearts and lungs. There were heads and torsos, and one with a double snake for the removal of curses and spells. I was not clear what happened to them after they were bought, whether they were offered in the sacred tank, or placed in the *samadhi*, but I was later told the amulets would be given to a priest, for a prayer to be said over them.

Sacred Garden. A sacred garden lay behind the tombs, in which only men were allowed to go. Two men cared for the plants (one had come as a patient ten years earlier). Men carried water from the well inside the garden in plastic containers to the *samadhi* area. Many herbs grown there were offered to people who were mentally ill. A paste made from herbs was plastered over the skulls of the mentally distressed at night, so they received healing energy of plants during sleep. The paste was then washed off in the morning.

A decoction was also made out of plants for the patients. It had medicinal properties and was imbued with 'grace' from the garden. Inside the garden was a large water jar containing a green coloured decoction, made of all the medicinal herbs. A glass was given to patients, offering healing properties of herbs in the garden. Women who required it were given a glass to drink outside the garden gate, but they were not allowed inside. Only flowers from this garden were allowed into the *samadhi*, no other flowers went inside.

Healing ritual. When we arrived at the Darga (shrine), my colleague and I sat within the brightly lit chamber by the *samadhi*. Then he was led into the tomb to perform a ritual, for only men were allowed. Inside he put the footprints of the saint on his head, and bought a green cloth to place over the tomb as part of the prayer. There was one particular Hindu family of the Vaiysha caste, coming from Palini and Pillai, whose duty it was to put the sacred cloth *'chadr'* over the *samadhi*. While he was there, I was led to one side of the chamber where a guide chanted a prayer over me and patted my head vigorously with a peacock feather fan. Apparently this was to strike out any evil spirits lurking within my person.

Later beside the *samadhi*, I was blessed again, drank holy water, and this time my head was brushed three times to shock out any residual spirits, to drive out entities and any evil influences that might have been with me.

Seated within the brightly lit outer tiled chamber were several trinket sellers with their wares on coloured blankets on the ground. There was a book of donations for pilgrims who gave thousands of rupees to the shrine. We saw huge wads of money change hands: enormous sums were collected and put into a safe. In the evening at 10pm there was a flurry of activity. Curtains were drawn across all the samadhi. Uniformed guards began closing and locking the inner gates. Those reading the Koran or sitting in silent prayer left. Some youths rushed in to kiss the threshold of the shrine before the last gate was closed, and we were all escorted out of the one unlocked gate into the sleeping halls beyond.

The atmosphere in the halls was dark with low lighting. It was in this area those who were mentally distressed resided during their stay at the mosque. In one particular area there were large round columns, in which thick iron chains were embedded. This was where the mentally ill had been chained, before the fire that led to the government banning all chaining. Only six or eight columns had iron rings, the rest were free.

Relatives brought patients with mental distress here, and stayed with them to look after them. They bathed in the water tank then went to the shrine. These days because of the fire in Chennai there were many fewer patients. Here in the sleeping hall, pilgrims camped and slept amongst graves of long dead people. Hundreds of people stayed in the immediate columned hall, and perhaps thousands more in the surrounding *mandapas* and raised plinths, which were constructed within one of the seven gates to the *samadhi*. In the centre of this hall of humanity was a man with a huge metal brazier, an industrial sized incense burner two-foot in diameter. He was fanning incense on red-hot coals, fanning a potent mixture over resting pilgrims, so the incense would lift any attached afflictions, curses or spirits. I gave him some rupees. I didn't want to attract any unnecessary attention in this place.

The following morning we walked by the water tank. It was a huge cement and stone construction, with separate bathing areas for men and women (the men having to pass through the woman's entrance in order to reach their own). In the tank, people made offerings of their hair. They had it clipped at the barbers', then when they were completely shaved they covered their skull with sandal paste. Their hair clippings were placed in a soft bread roll, and thrown into the tank as a votive offering. We watched as a pilgrim threw a bun, and the water boiled and churned as shoals of fish began frenzied feeding. The act of clipping one's hair, and putting it in a bread role was one stage in the process of making a wish or request at the mosque.

SUMMARY

We had visited religious institutions in Tamil Nadu, places which were renowned for alleviating mental distress. I'd travelled with Tamil speaking colleagues who kindly gave their time and the head priest from a Sri Murugan temple in London. We'd engaged in religious healing rituals ourselves and observed the daily practices of others, perambulating around multiple levels of temple precincts.

Dr Basu had come on one journey, seen local rituals, and made suggestions for incorporating psychiatric strategies with the religious practices. I discovered he was in the process of designing a healing centre in Pondicherry that addressed the ideas of Sri Aurobindo. He worked with architects and was expecting the plans to materialise and manifest.

During this trip, it became obvious to me, that people made pilgrimages to temples, churches and mosques, not only if they were distressed, but also for prophylactic purposes. In this way, they maintained mental peace in their daily lives. With this in mind, we decided to make a pilgrimage around religious and spiritual places, to discover what rituals seekers practiced for their mental well being. It felt inappropriate to focus only on strategies for addressing mental distress, when strategies for achieving mental peace were so much a part of normal practice in India. In the next chapter, we are joined again by one priest and his family from a London temple, who escorted us around Hindu temples in Tamil Nadu.

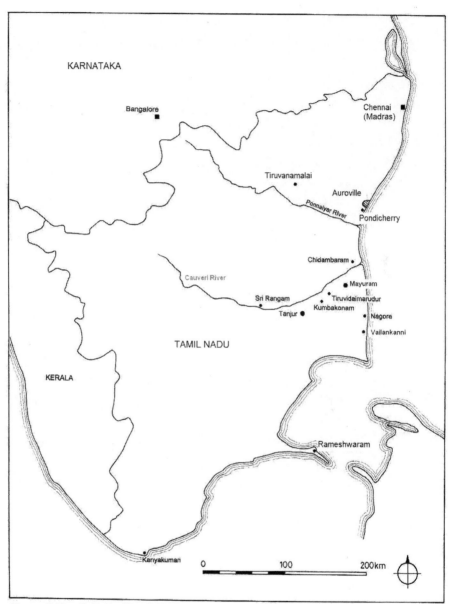

Figure 6 South India, Tamil Nadu

Chapter Seven

RELIGIOUS AND SPIRITUAL ESTABLISHMENTS FOR MENTAL PEACE

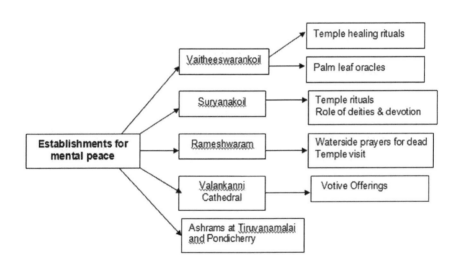

Introduction

This chapter presents sites which were renowned for providing mental peace to pilgrims. I visited a temple of healing at Vaitheeswarankoil, where there were libraries of ancient palm leaf oracles. Visitors inquired of these to enhance their mental peace, and a rich town had developed around the viewings.

Other sites visited include the temple at Rameshwaram, and the Cathedral to Our Lady at Vailankanni. Pilgrims went there to take *darshan* (to take sight of the deity). Since planetary influences were considered to be so important for mental peace, I visited several places that were crucial for pilgrims, and I have given a map (Figure 7) of the main planetary shrines in Tamil Nadu. The journeys made to the various establishments below were made from my base at Pondicherry, where I stayed in different guest houses over the time of the research.

The following establishments for finding mental peace were visited, and are mentioned in the texts below:
- Sri Vaidhyanatha Swami temple, Vaitheeswarankoil
- Vaitheeswarankoil, Palm Leaf Oracles
- Suryanakoil, temple to the nine planets
- Sri Ramanathaswamy temple, Rameshwaram
- Basilica to Our Lady of Health, Vailankanni Cathedral
- Ramana Maharshi Ashram at Tiruvannamalai
- Sri Aurobindo Ashram at Pondicherry

Religious Establishments for Mental Peace

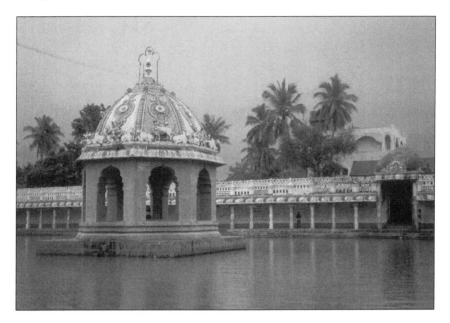

Water tank at Vaitheeswarankoil temple

Vaitheeswarankoil: Sri Vaidhyanathaswami temple

We visited the town of Vaitheeswarankoil with Naganathan, head priest of the Sri Murugan temple in East London, UK. We were told men and women who were considered possessed could remove the possessing spirits by bathing in the tank of the Sri Vaidhyanatha Swami temple.

We entered the temple complex through a walled rectangular water tank, with stepped sides, and a walkway right around it. This was the Siddhamirtham Thirtha, governed by saint Dhanavanti, who was Lord of Medicine and resided below the waters in the area of the central domed *mandapa*. Every pilgrim bathed in the waters of the tank before going through the temple entrance, or at least they washed their hands and feet. Student physicians were encouraged to visit this temple before exams.

The water was teeming with shoals of large fish, which were over a foot long. It was said that if a person with a skin disorder bathed in the water, and was touched by the fish, which gently bit their limbs, they became cured[44]. After bathing at this stepped tank, we walked around, to the left, and into the temple entrance, opposite the tank entrance. My colleague (a junior physician) and I followed three procedures for health and peace of mind: dissolving sugar cane in the water of the tank; making prayers at five different shrines; and finally having a private prayer with a priest who offered a medicine pellet that would protect us from physical and mental ill health.

This wealthy temple complex was around 11 acres, with inscriptions dating from 12th century AD[45]. It was where Shiva was renowned as a physician and herbalist. The presiding deity was Sri Vaidhyanatha Swami, the healer of all diseases and the place was governed by the planet Mars. The western *gopura* (tower) was constructed in such a way that at a certain time of year, the sun's rays passed through it and fell directly onto the lingam in the central shrine. Within the complex was a large margosa tree (*melia azadirachta*) of great sanctity, claimed to have powerful medicinal properties.

Healing Rituals. A guide took us around and led us through the first three rituals. In order to wash away our sins *(dosha)* from this life and any previous ones, we followed certain proscribed rituals. First we made devotions to Ganapathi. Then we took some palm sugar (*jaggery*) and dissolved it in the waters of the tank with our right hand. As this votive offering dissolved, all our physical ailments dissolved with it. We were told those who took a full dip in the waters, would never get ill again. We cupped water in our hands and offered it three times to the head of the *shiva lingam* on a column at the water's edge. And then did *pranam* (obeisance) with our hands clasped.

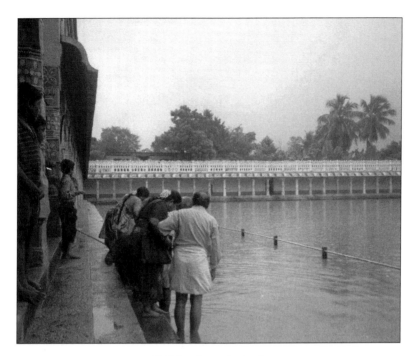

Bathing in water tank

The offering of water was a gesture of surrendering our problems to Shiva. The flowers we placed on the column were symbols of perfection. We were given two little sachets of salt and pepper, which we offered in order to clear any skin diseases. We each broke the sachets into a huge container, then our attendant gave us a few grains of salt and one peppercorn to eat. We had completed the first stage of rituals.

We undertook the second stage of rituals with a priest (*pujari*). Our guide introduced us to a young priest, with a whitened face and the marks of Shiva in sacred ash on his forehead, arms and rounded belly. He had trained in computer technology, and worked in the temple because his father had worked there before him. He took our names and prayed all our past sins would be removed. He wore one gold amulet around his neck, as well as a *rudraksha* bead on a thread. Taking us around various inner shrines, he recited mantras while we each held an offering basket, which the guide had prepared. As he chanted our names, plus the names of our immediate family, his voice rang out clearly at each shrine. There were five main deities, and we stood directly in front of the shrines of each in order to receive *darshan*, or catch their 'eye'. This was considered extremely healing.

The attendant priests at the shrines were all barefoot and bare-chested, wearing lunghi and a single thread around their shoulders to their waist. Some wore jewellery, such a diamond in one ear, or gold rings. We walked in a single file, in a clockwise direction, right around the back of each shrine.

We were joined by members of Naganathan's family, and after paying ten rupees 'special entrance' we sat by the shrine of Subramanya, which was crowded with pilgrims. A row of priests on either side of the entrance chanted mantras, and the sound was huge and magnificent. We arrived in time to see the anointing ceremony of the main deity, who was covered with yoghurt. When it was wiped away from his eyes, the crowd roared in ecstasy as the priests lifted the flames to allow us to be seen by the deity's eyes (*darshan*). Devotees near me slapped their cheeks with their palms or hit their foreheads with closed fists three times, as part of their request for all their sins to be absolved. We received the flame from the inner sanctum, put it over our eyes and were given a pinch of sacred ash. At each shrine we put ash afresh on our foreheads and collected sacred ash and vermilion in tiny pinches in tiny paper packets to take back home. It was sanctified since it had been in front of the deity. We were given petals and sacred leaves too, flowers to put in our hair, and roses.

People came to this temple to gain will power. The rituals here were particularly good for people affected by the negative influences of the planet Mars. In the area of the Navagrahas, the nine planets were set in a single line, facing the main deity, so they could each see him at once. Passing before the planets set out in this configuration was itself healing, since it released any karmic-carryover a person was born with. Here, unusually the moon was given considerable importance being the deity with influence over our emotions. It was placed even higher than the sun. We walked by the images of the deities of the nine planets, to release any planetary karmic influence, which we were born with that might be affecting our own health. In one corridor, there were 108 *shiva lingams*, with the deity of Surya (the sun) standing by in supporting role.

During the third stage of rituals, the priest conducted a private ceremony, with us seated in a circle on the ground around him, outside the shrine of Parvati (consort of Shiva). He said prayers and offered us some sandal wood paste mixed with saffron, over which priests had chanted prayers. We applied this to our foreheads in order to have success in any endeavour.

We were given a tiny round pill, in our right hand, like a homoeopathic pill, which we had to swallow immediately. I though it tasted gritty as if made of ash and sand. In fact it was rolled from mud from the water tank mixed with *vibhuti* (sacred ash) from a shrine that had been offered in pellet form to Thaiyalnayaki, consort of the Lord of Medicine. It incorporated the following ingredients: bilwa leaf, nim leaf, sandal paste, vibhuti, soil from the temple garden. This was prepared as a paste in rose water. By consuming the rounded pellets, we removed any diseases within. These pellets had been made from a recipe given by Lord Dhanavanti, god of physicians, with Shiva the Master Physician. All medicines came from this source. There was a garden behind the temple, which was hidden from view and only the person who worked in it was permitted to gather the ingredients there. No priests were allowed in.

In each shrine we had to wait while the priest said some mantras at the inner sanctum. He lit a square of camphor, waved it in front of the deities, then brought it out to us, where we moved our hands over it, and accepted an offering of *vibhuti* (ash) and vermillion. The priest offered the deity the flower garlands, coconut, camphor and *vibhuti*. We ended the ritual by leaving money on the tray, and taking the flowers, fruit and coconut wrapped in a plastic bag. Then we gave the priest some money gifts in exchange for accompanying us. These prayers and rituals should have cleared up any melancholy held within myself from then onwards. I was hopeful.

Vaitheeswarankoil: Palm Leaf Oracles

I returned later with a colleague Dr Mohan to the town of Vaitheeswarankoil where there were numerous Astrology offices, and many places to see palm leaf oracles, and receive a personal interpretation. The oracles brought a sense of mental peace to many people. They confirmed the client was on the right track in life, and offered suggestions for what to do about problems if there were any. We went into one astrologer's offices, though I couldn't face having another reading, after all the unsolicited information I had been given earlier during my stay, but I wanted to photograph a palm leaf.

Vaitheeswarankoil was the main town for palm leaf readings (or *nadi*), though there were branch libraries in Kumbakonam and Chennai. The 15th century monastery at Thiruvavaduthurai contained 1,200 bundles, inscribed using a stylus[46]. The palm leaves were written 'thousands' of years ago by Sanskrit scholars, and were translated into Tamil. There were several 'libraries' in the town where the bundles were kept. At first only two or three families were involved in interpretation, but by 2003 more than 30 families did readings. The town appeared to be wealthy with many new hotels.

I interviewed Dr Mohan who had visited astrologers in this town. The first time he came out of curiosity: he had heard how surprised people were when they found out everything about them had already been written down. He was concerned readers or 'astrologers' may misread or select a wrong leaf. *"What I found was during the readings that they said things to please you whatever was written. They were interpreting things on their own which they had not got from the palm leaves"*. Although he said *"I have faith in the palm leaves themselves. I have faith in the wisdom of the rishis who lived thousands of years ago, who had seen things and written them down"*.

The palm leaf readers and interpreters are known by the generic term 'astrologer' which means anything from psychic to clairvoyant, seer to intuitive to palm reader. Successful readers became very wealthy with funds received from satisfied clients. *"Now it is very commercialised here and whether you are rich or poor you have to pay the same money. That is the sad part of the place, where some of the wisdom has been commercialised. It is a wisdom that doesn't belong to them, but to the rishis, who were never commercial."*

The second time the doctor chose a different reader. He was in the middle of his professional career, under some stress, not sure which direction to take, and not sure what the future held. He also had personal issues he wanted to resolve. *"It was not clear where my life was leading, whether I was doing the right thing, or just following my whim, or whether I was doing God's wish, or what was destined for me…. I just wanted to have confirmation and to know whether I was on the right path."*

In the palm leaf oracles, there were fourteen or fifteen general *kandams* (or chapters). They were divided into different subject matter: one for your past lives, one for the sins of your past lives (*dosha*), one for all the prayers and rituals you should do, and a separate one for the chances you have. There were separate ones for your problems and your family, your marriage, and for professional life. There was one for all the chronic diseases humans had, and ways to get rid of them. The doctor explained "*Only the person whose palm leaf is there will come, and he will only come at a particular time in his life. So it is already destiny when you go there and when you find your leaf. There must be wisdom behind it.*"

During an appointment, a client's right thumb-print was taken. Based on the print, its matching lines and spots, the appropriate bundle of palm leaves was found. With one or two questions, the readers would determine whether they had the correct leaf. Once this was found, they wrote down the information and interpreted it for the client. I asked the doctor what he gained from having the readings. "*I felt that even thousands of years ago it was already planned that I would come at this particular time, in this particular century, to this particular family, bearing this particular name, and having this particular profession, and I'll be going in this particular direction. If we ignore the commercial part of it then it is very beautiful. It was not a simple astrological prediction.*"

It was widely believed everything was written on the palm leaves, and they were not only appropriate for people in India, but beyond. Once a reading had taken place, prayer rituals required should be carried out in the appropriate places: the palm leaves indicated the temples and rituals that were necessary. Visitors went there because of the Navagraha temples, the temples to the nine planets, like Suryanarkoil described below, which were all situated in this region.

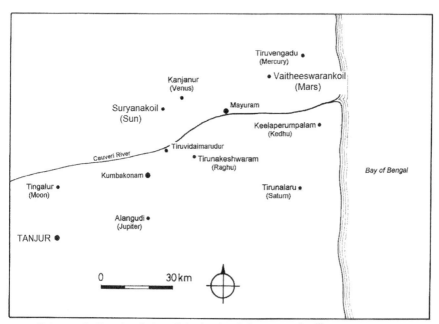

Figure 7 Navagraha Temples, that mediate planetary influences on health

Suryanarkoil: temple to the nine planets

I remembered the temple of Suryanarkoil in Tanjur District as a small pleasant place, painted in yellow with beautifully decorated sculptures. When we arrived this time, the surrounding streets were crowded with cars. It was Sunday, the day of the sun, and everyone had come to Suryanarkoil (temple of the sun) in order to worship and perform rituals. The sun deity liked the colour red, and so many people had brought him red flowers.

Dr Basu had told me planetary influences affected his patients' well being. For example, on the day of the dark moon (no moon day), many people tried to kill themselves. He had lots of cases of attempted suicide on days of no moon and full moon. This particular Shiva temple at Suryanarkoil was where the nine planets granted a boon: those who prayed here should not be affected by trials and tribulations of planetary influences. It was said people would be relieved of their maladies and afflictions when they worshipped here. They would be absolved of all their sins and diseases. Propitiating the planets was said to bring peace of mind, reduce mental tension, and allow mental agonies to ease[47].

At the entrance people were buying nine tiny ceramic lamps, filled with a wick and a little cream coloured wax. First they received blessings from the main deity, the sun. In this position the sun could reduce or annul the influence of Saturn, which affected physical and mental ailments. This temple was the only one dedicated to all nine planets. The main deity in the inner sanctum was the sun, and all the other planets had their own separate shrines located outside in the temple courtyard. The pilgrims visited each in a clockwise perambulation and offered a lamp at each.

When the world was created, it was said, first there was the sound 'AUM', and from that sound, the sun appeared. At this temple, planets appeared in their benevolent form, and they did not hold any weapons. For people who performed the procedure of worshipping the sun, this removed mental worries, especially if it was done on a Sunday. The tree outside the shrine in the courtyard was hung with cloths. After prayer these were hung in order to remove a person's sins from previous incarnations. There was also a temple to the moon at Thirujalur. Pilgrims who visited this one got relief from mental distress. On Mondays, people worshiped using white flowers.

Role of deities & devotion. I asked Dr Loganathan, the medical herbalist I'd met earlier, to explain the role of deities and devotion. I hadn't fully understood his argument that deities were not worshipped as idols in themselves, but each one was linked to a particular planet. Thus by worshipping the deities, one was creating a relationship with other aspects of the planetary universe and the cosmos. He said: *"planets are linked to the different gods and goddess that people worship. Shiva is the creator of the sun. People cannot worship the sun every day in the morning, but they can worship Shiva every day in the temple, and like all planets, Shiva, Parvati, Lakshmi, Murugan, Mahavishnu, Brahma, Ulligamma and Kali, these are all the reflections of the different planets".*

I asked whether this was like a vibrational link, whether devotees thought they were looking at Saraswathi, but she was linked with a particular planet. *"Yes and so by worshipping Ganesh and Murugan, you are worshipping Mars. It is not well understood by the people, and that is why it is very important. In ancient times we were understanding problems of how to take things to the grass roots level. We know the sun is responsible for all kinds of energy, and also its importance for us living in this world".*

"But the problem is how to feed this knowledge and information to people at grass roots level, to the lay person living in a village with a different exposure. Perhaps by saying Shiva is linked to the sun god, that he created this world and protects it and destroys it. Shiva has all these qualities. We say you must worship Shiva, then you are protecting your family, environment and nature. In that way people understand it. That is how this kind of worship of images arises. If on that level when they want to develop, then they can adapt. It is not just Shiva, with one head or two heads or three heads. It is not that, it is linked to this planet, which is responsible for the world's living and survival".

This was the first time I had understood the ancient role of deity worship described like this, as a means of connecting with planetary energies in the universe. Dr Loganathan's perspective on the role of deities and planets was more profound that I had heard before. The simple worship of idols was a way of linking with the planets within the universe. With much to reflect on, my companion and I continued on our way: our next journey was to Rameshwaram on the coast of Tamil Nadu.

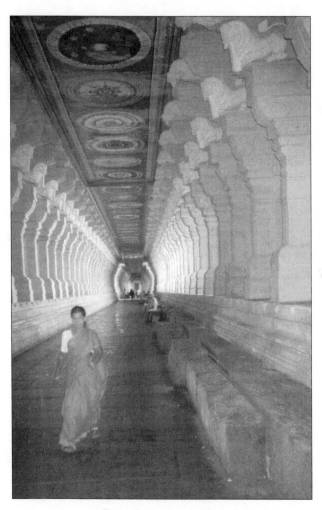

Rameshwaram corridors

Rameshwaram Ramanathaswamy temple

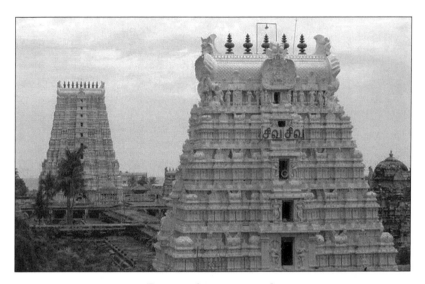

Ramanathaswamy temple

There were said to be four energy points in India, which held the soul of the continent and the people together. One of these sites was at Rameshwaram. If in their lifetime, someone went to all four places, they were certain to have a connection to their soul. However, if they did not do it, then they would have to incarnate for many life times before the opportunity would be provided again. Of all these energy points, Rameshwaram was the only Shaivite temple: the others were Vaishnava. It was considered to be the Benares of the south, and was used by both followers of Shiva and Vishnu as a place of worship.

The temple complex covered 15.5 acres. The presiding deity was Sri Ramanathaswamy, Sri Rama Lingam[48]. It was associated with the Ramayana epic, and was where Rama worshipped Siva to expiate his sin of having killed Ravanna. There were 22 sacred wells within the temple, and bathing in them in sequence "purifies the body and the soul"[49], and purified oneself of one's sins. Legend had it that Lord Rama himself had installed the lingam there.

Prayer rituals for the dead. The sea front at Rameshwaram was a place for prayers for the dead, a place where rituals were conducted for mental peace, and for closure after bereavement. My colleague and I arrived late one evening. Hundreds of coaches, cars, and trucks were parked on waterfront roads, decorated with garlands of yellow marigolds. That day hundreds of Ayyappa pilgrims had come: they incorporated this town as part of their pilgrimage route. Bathing in the sea here was said to absolve all one's sins, and to be very purifying. On the sea-front there was an elderly government worker in a khaki uniform, collecting cloths, and pulling hundreds of black dhoti out of the sand. He made a huge pile of these black cloths and other clothes each day, which pilgrims discarded as they plunged into the sea. People were taking photographs of each other in the water or on the rocks. There were professional photographers, local boys with Polaroid cameras strapped around their necks, offering quick photos. Rows of beggars lined the road.

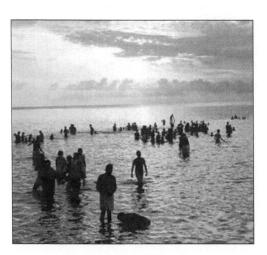

Dawn Bathing at Rameshwaram

The following morning at 6am, we stood at the sea front. There were thousands of men, dressed in black robes, thousands on the seashore, with black eyes, black hair, black beards, and black *dhotis*. They strode into the sea in groups and ducked their heads under the water. These were the Ayyappa, stripping down to their under garments and underpants then going out to sea in a group. Once they reached the seashore, they flung their dhotis into the water.

Further down the beach, in a quieter area, men were squatting on their buttocks defecating into the water, and afterwards washing their hands and nether regions with sea water. Others were cleaning their teeth, with foaming froth, and rinsing their mouths in seawater. One man had a toothpaste foam trail dripping on his huge round belly.

There were women fully clothed in their saris, dipping into the sea. We stood there for a long time, perhaps four or five hours, just watching. I stood amongst this seething throng of humans, cows and crows. Nobody noticed me, and it felt wonderful, as if I was invisible. Later, when I got my photos back I saw why. I stood amongst the crowd with a cow beside me. With the shawl covering my head, and wearing a brown *salwa khamis*, perhaps people thought I was a pale pilgrim from the north?

The seashore beside the temple at Rameshwaram was a place to perform ceremonies for the mental peace of both the living and the dead. Pilgrims came with the ashes of deceased relatives, and offered them to the waters. Ashes were brought in little ceramic pots, which after a ceremony were taken into the sea with an offering of fresh flower garlands. On the shore there were a number of freelance pundits (brahmin pujaris) pitched up on the sands, sitting under umbrellas, with the full paraphernalia of their trade laid out in front of them. Each dealt with people from a particular part of India, so they would perform the ceremony pertinent to their own customs and rituals. They specialised in one geographical area, offering prayers for the dead for specific castes.

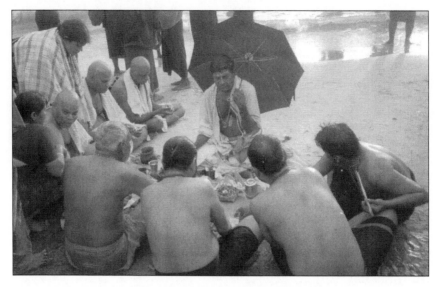

Pundit's service for bereaved families

One priest sat cross-legged on the sand just in front of me, sheltered from the light drizzle by an umbrella. He was performing ceremonies to two sets of people simultaneously. Sitting beside him were three brothers with shaved heads and thick-set features. (In the south it was the custom for all brothers to shave their heads on the death of a parent, whereas in the north, only the eldest shaved.) In front of them there was a dark brown ceramic pot with a lid containing the ashes of their father. The ashes in the pot received an anointing *(abishekam)* of milk, poured from a steel teacup. Each of the brothers was given some rice paste, with which they made twelve or thirteen small balls, about an inch in diameter. Then their father's ashes were incorporated into these small rice balls, laid on a raft of long grasses *(dharba)*, and embellished with flower petals.

This area attracted many cows and unfortunately one started eating the rice balls before ceremonial prayers had been said. Female members of the family tried to move the cow away, but it had already consumed a great deal. The other brothers took their balls of rice and put them on concrete posts by the roadside. From here it was appropriate for the calves and cows to eat, and they moved in and consumed them immediately. Above us, perched on the electricity wires, sat dozens of chattering crows also waiting for their share.

Once the rice balls had been placed, the three brothers walked three times around the pundits, then the eldest took the little pot of ashes upon his head, and followed by the other two, he walked into the sea, as far as he could go. Then they let seawater fill the pot, and offered it into the sea. The ceramic pot and its contents were gifted into the sea, followed by a garland of fresh flowers. As we watched the flowers drifting into the ocean, they stood with their hands together in *pranayam,* for long minutes in total stillness. Wearing white dhoti, they undid the cloth, allowing the sea to take that away, until they stood in just underclothes. A dozen other family members with the three brothers, then had brief words with the pundit and walked ceremonially around him.

Further down the shore, one woman walked out alone into the sea, fully clothed in her deep purple sari. She let the sea take her little ceramic pot, and all its contents. After it was carried away, she ducked herself completely under the water. These rituals were conducted for mental peace and for closure after bereavement. Many people brought their relatives' ashes here. By evening the sea shore was littered again with thousands of *dhotis* and other clothes, trodden into the sand or caught between the rocks. Then the government employee in the khaki uniform collected all the cloths and put them in a pile by the rocks. By that evening the clothes mountain was over a meter high.

Taking waters of the 22 wells. The following morning my colleague and I visited the shrines of the Ramanathaswamy Temple. It seemed as though the walls and long corridors of the temple were shouting out with the sounds of hundreds of years of memory. The stone floors were soaking wet and slippery underfoot. It was the custom for pilgrims to bathe at first light in the sea, the men wearing simple dhotis, young children naked, older ones around seven or eight in their underwear, and the women in their saris. All were soaked to the skin and dripping, the women clutching the men's arms to stop themselves from slipping. It was most auspicious to do this pilgrimage as a couple.

At each well the guide would draw up a bucket, and pour water over each pilgrim's head. The waters from the wells were said to have medicinal properties, they refreshed the mind, and gave relief from mental agony[50]. They were also used to ward off one's sins and to remove insanity. We were told bathing in water from the wells allowed our minds to become sane. Escorted by our guide, we completed all 22 wells, then visited other nearby shrines on the peninsula.

At Rameshwaram, we took a horse and cart taxi and went up the hill to visit shrines outside the town. At one a priest offered to perform perfunctory prayers for money, with little or no religiosity attached. In others it was a similar story, prayers for money, a few words mumbled, the wave of a lighted lamp, a pinch of ash and vermilion, and a coin or note in exchange. I became exhausted by these flat religious rituals, performed for visiting pilgrims. I did not want to visit anywhere else that day: we left and returned to the hotel.

Vailankanni Cathedral

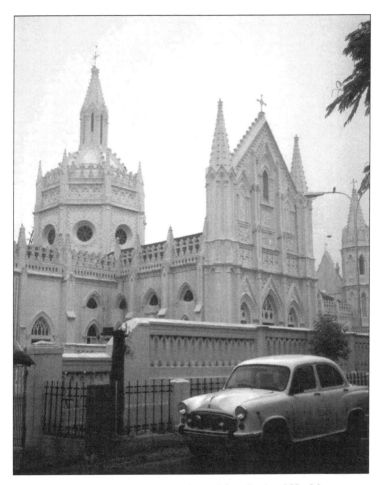

Vailankanni Shrine Basilica of Our Lady of Health

The following week, we drove further along the coast of the Bay of Bengal to Vailankanni Cathedral, a Basilica to Our Lady of Health. It stood like an elegant iced-gateau against the sky. This was a place people came to achieve mental and physical peace. Like the mosque at Nagore described earlier, it welcomed people of all faiths to receive its healing powers. There were thousands of pilgrims during festival times, and as we had arrived on Christmas Eve, the roads were crowded to capacity. Inside the Basilica was swept spotlessly clean. There was not even a grain of sand on the floor. Pilgrims sat in prayer, in front of the shrine of Our Lady. The paintings over the shrine were in beautiful blues and pinks, surrounded by an arc of angels. Our Lady was covered in thick garlands of flowers, in reds, yellows and white. A group of women quietly sang hymns: there was an atmosphere of peace, as people queued up to make offerings of flowers, coconuts and candles.

Walking down the lane to the seafront, we noticed shops were selling hundreds of effigies. These were in white wax, and included body parts, organs, arms and legs, whole human beings, babies, boys and girls. They were also heads (about 10cms high) for those suffering from mental ailments. It was the custom to take the wax head and give it in as an offering at the side entrance of the church, from where it would be taken and put in front of Our Lady.

Votive Offerings. Inside the cathedral's neighbouring museum, we walked through row after a row of display cases. Each housed votive offerings in gold or silver, sent in by pilgrims to express thanks for a wish granted, whether it was for health, wealth, profession, or offspring. There were hundreds of tiny cots, houses in silver sheeting, whole ships, engineer's tools, doctor's paraphernalia and a car mechanic's equipment. There were also many health related items including an elaborate pair of lungs, a huge heart, limbs and body organs. The letters accompanying the offerings gave testament to miracles of health, which had occurred with or without the use of bio-medicine. Some prayers were from people whose tumours or diseases had been spontaneously cured, and they offered thanks because they hadn't needed invasive medicine. A few were in English, the rest in Tamil. The priest we spoke to said about half the people who came were Christian, half were Hindu, and there was a handful of Muslims.

Legend claimed towards the end of 16th or early 17th century, Mary the mother of Jesus appeared in the small fishing village of Vailankanni. She appeared to a young boy selling milk under a Banyan tree: he had never seen anything like it, and was filled with awe. The first chapel was built after Mother Mary saved some seafarers from death, and bought their boat ashore there[51]. Lying in the Bay of Bengal, a few kilometres from Nagore, it was known as "the Lourdes of the Orient".

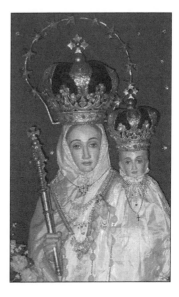

Our Lady of Health

At the time of its origin the land belonged to the Vijayanagara empire, and was referred to in literary sources in 1630 AD. Even today many visions and apparitions continue to appear to people. In 2002 the inhabitants, including the floating population, numbered some 30,000.

The head priest saw himself as an administrator: he collected pilgrims' offerings sent in after successful prayers, and suggested some for display. His desk was full of paperwork. All day long people queued at his door and he blessed them with water from a long-necked silver vessel. He clearly felt he himself played no part in the healing process.

People prayed directly to Our Lady of Health, and received direct miracles. He repeatedly said he played no role in any miracles, and the church did not play a role in mental health: there were no psychiatric patients there. However, he said there was nothing to stop people coming themselves with the mentally ill, and praying directly. However in 1998, the church established a school for learning disability children.

It was said Mother Mary *"repairs broken bodies, mends torn hearts, and restores skin and sacred souls"*[52]. They were so many votive offerings that the cathedral had to build a special hall to house them. The museum halls provided 'living testimony of God's providence through Mary'[53] and all the offerings were from those who had experienced divine intervention. Within the shrine there was a belief spiritual events could not be bought or sold by intermediaries: prayer was by direct application only. The shrine authorities built many sleeping halls (*mandapa*) for the pilgrims of many different faiths who visited, and who were helped by Mary during their stay on earth. That evening we drove back northwards along the coast to the seafront town of Pondicherry.

Ashrams for Mental Peace

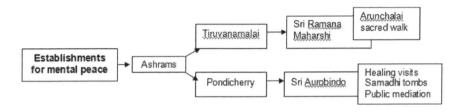

Sri Ramana Maharshi's ashram, Tiruvanamalai

Several weeks later I caught the train from Pondicherry railway station with my travelling companion, and we visited the ashram of Sri Ramana Maharshi at Tiruvanamalai, a few hours away. The sage Sri Ramana Maharshi died in 1950 the same year as Sri Aurobindo. This calm ashram was set in beautiful gardens, where peacocks and mischievous monkeys roamed freely. We arrived late, and as the sun went down, monkeys came into the garden to play, wildly leaping from the trees onto the building and jumping onto the barred windows.

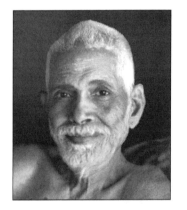

As dusk fell, peacocks flew up to the tall treetops, to spend the night. Set at the foothills of the sacred Mountain Arunachala, there were numerous rooms where pilgrims seeking mental peace, could stay.

Sri Ramana Maharshi

This ashram attracted huge crowds, and hundreds of westerners. Some had moved into lodgings in the town, and made it their home. Here was a younger hippie looking crowd wearing multi coloured clothing: some women wore Indian dress, a sari or *salwa khamis*; some wore tight T-shirts with no bras, with flowers in their hair, and others carried babies. The men looked young, cheerful and carefree, with shaggy hair and long beards, or dread locks. They drank fruit juice at the bars, and ate chocolate cake and cinnamon biscuits at German cafes. There were also older westerners: women with well-groomed cropped hair, and designer painted saris. One, who looked like a fashion model, had finely styled blonde hair, wore a long turquoise skirt, a purple T-shirt, and a deep blue shawl.

That evening many foreigners sat quietly against the marble walls of the meditation room. In the central chamber, priests continuously chanted over the *samadhi*. In the hall adjoining the temple it was the custom to walk around the central *samadhi*, in a clockwise direction. People walked singly, seriously, doing a meditative walk. Sometimes devotees prostrated themselves on the ground, lying belly down, with arms outstretched. Some knelt and placed their foreheads on the ground. There were notices up, warning people not to carry valuables with them while meditating: theft of personal belongings was a concern. Next to the great hall with the *samadhi* was a Hindu temple, where *pujaris* administered prayers. A side room, the Maharishi's own room, was always full of people in meditation. On the bed on which he lay, was a four foot painting of him reclining on that same bed with the table lamp beside him.

The entire area of *Arunachala Hill* was considered sacred, the embodiment of Shiva, so it was the pilgrims' practise to walk barefoot to the cave where the Maharishi lived from 1900 to 1916, and then onto Bhavan shrine (Skandashram) where he spent time from 1916 to 1922. The following morning my travelling companion and I followed a path up and around the hill covered with pink granite rounded boulders. Spiritual pilgrims came to this hill from all over the world: the Japanese wore white clothes and carried umbrellas to protect them from the hot sun.

On the path we met a wandering *sadu*, a holy man in his 50's, with a round face, a stocky well-fed body and dark skin. He wore a white dhoti and bright red cloth around his middle. Across his shoulders he carried a white cloth bag, with all his possessions. He slept in the hills. His face was benevolent and looked munificent. This wandering sadu called himself Maheshwara. He calmly asked whether we had time in our busy schedules to talk with him. My companion sat on a boulder beside him to chat, looking pale, thin, and not fully embodied. He asked the *sadu* about the meaning of life, the soul, the body, the purpose of realisation, and the point of being in a human body. The sage answered questions in a quiet voice, so low we had to strain to hear it, even in the silence of the hills. When he had finished talking, he invited us to continue on our way.

We walked up to the first small Bhavan shrine, the place where the saint stayed until 1922, where plastic rush mats were laid out around the walls. Pilgrims, mostly westerners, but not all, were meditating in a state of calm serenity. Holy water from the inner hill was supplied by hosepipe down to a tap from which one could drink. There were trees and green plants growing in this cool oasis of calm. I sat inside the shrine and felt as if I had the hands of the saint on my belly, healing old wounds. I felt as if I glowed with light. Later we sat on a rocky out crop high up on the hill, with a view over the city and its huge temple walkways, filled with trees. As we sat eight hawks flew all around us, so close we could hear the air on their wings, and the swirling energy around us, above us, and beneath us, lower down the hill.

We walked on to Venkatesh cave where the sage spent time from 1900 until 1916. A notice said he built the inner platforms himself. Deep within this bouldered cave, now painted white throughout, was an earthen *shiva lingam* and a single flame.

People sat silently inside, one person read quietly. There were a number of pictures of Sri Ramana Maharshi lining the walls, each at different ages, different poses, always wearing just a simple loin cloth, his eyes in later years smiling with such benevolent compassion.

Later that evening, we joined hundreds of people sitting in rows in the dining hall, eating off fresh banana leaves, or small dried leaves stitched together to form a circular plate. Helpers served us: they ladled food out from aluminium buckets, quickly and efficiently, with several different vegetable combinations, plus rice, buttermilk and water in metal cups. On the walls, three rows deep, were many pictures of the Maharishi and other saints. In the bookshop, lining one wall was a calendar, which was spread along the upper walls, each month illustrating him in a different pose, like any western pop star calendar.

In the restaurant the next morning, by some curious coincidence, I was accosted by a *pujari*, a Hindu priest, with his long black hair in a bun on top of his head. He reminded me we had met earlier in London at another priest's house. His family home was in Tiruvanamalai and so he invited me there. He lived in a small house near the temple, and supported his wife, two sons and a daughter, and his sisters. He spent six months each year in UK, and six in India.

He worked in London as a freelance *pujari,* not attached to any temple, but travelling to wherever he was called to do prayers, whether it was Manchester or Malaysia. He said he did not want to be reborn, so he was prepared to fully experience anything life offered including any illness. In that way he would not need to take another rebirth. He had problems with his digestion, and now he could afford to eat nice food, his health wouldn't allow it. "*It's all karma*", he said gently, accepting his lot. My travelling companion and I thanked him for his hospitality and left Tiruvanamalai that afternoon to travel back to Pondicherry.

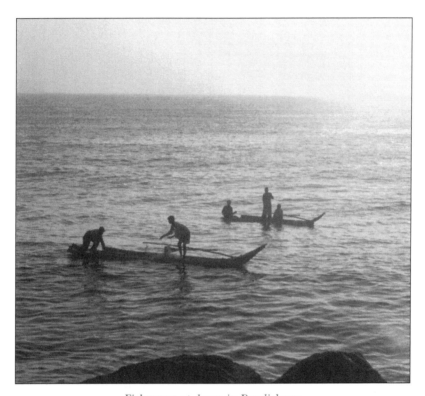

Fishermen at dawn in Pondicherry

Pondicherry, Sri Aurobindo Ashram

Pondicherry Sea Front. During my travels to religious and spiritual institutions across Tamil Nadu, I was based in a hotel in the town of Pondicherry. In the early mornings, people did exercises by the sea before the sun came up. The whole town seemed to walk along the beach promenade before dawn and every evening around dusk. They walked briskly for exercise before sunrise, doing yoga exercises and stretching. In the garden by Park Guest House where I stayed, sometimes groups of men did synchronised stretching movements together. Others sat cross-legged on the sea wall, gazing out across the vast expanse of ocean, waiting for the sun to rise.

On rainy days, men rode up and down the sea-road on their bicycles, holding an umbrella in one hand. One week it rained for three days. Torrential rain. The sky was dark and cloudy, and when the rain was not torrential, there was a continuous drizzle. The wind blew furiously. The sea air, sand and grit covered everything. My skin became sticky from the salt, my hair went frizzy, and my clothes were clammy. Even the bed sheets felt damp from the sea air. Perpetual damp.

The wind was relentless, so penetrating I could barely walk along the beachfront. The waves were furious: they smashed on the rocky sea walls of Pondicherry with such force, with such anger, all day and all night. Palm trees groaned and leant away from the wind.

Later that evening, the air became very still. It was cloudy, but dead still, there was no movement, no wind, the curtains in my room didn't even rustle. The sea was at peace. The calm was so calm, it felt unnatural. A great peace came over me. I went into the meditation room at the guesthouse, and sat in the white room with huge photos of Sri Aurobindo and the Mother, and felt very supported. It was as if there was an energy, an unseen force holding me. I envisioned a tall white column of light, which I interpreted as Sri Aurobindo's presence. I thought I saw Nasreen, my deceased friend, dancing in a western dress, her hands on my shoulders. I felt contained, calm, and blessed. I slept well that night.

The following day I woke at 4.00 am. My thoughts about the research tumbled out in different directions. I had given up trying to think in a linear manner. My brain simply wasn't available. By 4.30am I gave up trying to sleep, and got up to see the sun rise over the sea. Outside it was cold and windy and I walked up and down the beach front, along with thousands of other people. I watched the red sun rising, huge over the sea, fringed with gold. The sun rose late that day then quickly hid behind some clouds. Radiant sunlight shot out at bright angles into the sky. It was a marvellous sunrise, with golden sunrays radiating out from behind the clouds, which were deep purple below, white on top, with an edging of pink cloud fringed with light. It felt like a special day.

Sri Aurobindo

Sri Aurobindo came to live in Pondicherry in 1910, and spent the last 40 years of his life there. Born in 1872 in Calcutta, he was a revolutionary, poet and visionary. He was educated at St Paul's in London and King's College Cambridge. He participated in India's struggle for freedom, and became a leader of the nationalist movement. In 1908, while in solitary confinement, awaiting trial, accused of alleged terrorist activities against the British (for which he was subsequently acquitted), Sri Aurobindo began to receive inspirational insights. On his release in 1910 he withdrew from the political field, and came to live in Pondicherry, where he devoted himself to his spiritual mission. Silencing his mind, he received divine guidance about the nature of human existence, evolution on earth, and cosmic consciousness. He passed away in 1950.

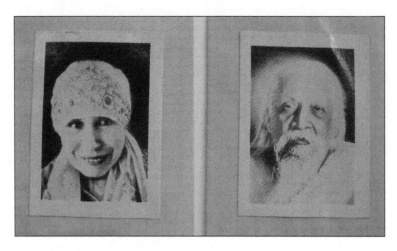

Mother and Sri Aurobindo

In 1914, Madame Mirra Alfassa, known as the Mother, joined Sri Aurobindo in this spiritual mission. Born in Paris in 1878, of a Turkish father and Egyptian mother, she had had unusual dreams and visions since she was a child. Like Sri Aurobindo, she was an inter-dimensional seer. In 1960 she founded the Sri Aurobindo Society to explore ways of looking inside oneself in order to solve the 'outer problems of human existence'. Her aim was to manifest Sri Aurobindo's vision: to create a society that embodied the new consciousness and included ideals about physical transformation. An ashram grew up around Sri Aurobindo and the Mother. This consisted of an international community whose members wanted to realise the visions in a practical manner. Their ideal was to achieve divine life on earth as part of physical existence.

The Society had over 300 centres throughout the world, and its charitable and research status was recognised by the Government of India. The ashram provided essential services and food for its members, and there were farms, handicraft and art centres, educational institutions and a gymnasium. It gave people housing, clothes, a bike, an umbrella every two years, it did the laundry for them and gave them a quota of food and flour. The intention was to develop all activities to help the growth of a new consciousness. Every year, certain events commemorating the life and times of Sri Aurobindo and the Mother were celebrated by followers, both at the ashram in Pondicherry, and at centres across the world. For public meditations, devotees sat either in the ashram or in the International Ashram School gardens.

Special Meditation: Sri Aurobindo's death anniversary. On 5th December, the day of Sri Aurobindo's death, his *mahasamadhi* (the day he left his body), I woke at 4.30am after hearing muffled noises in the corridor. I dressed and left for the ashram meditation while it was still dark. I found a place inside by the *samadhi (tomb)* with my back along the wall, next to elderly devotees, who also needed the wall for support. I sat in a corner by the plants, and felt comforted by the darkness. Gradually the place filled up, with elderly ladies and gentlemen brought in by their carers, in wheelchairs.

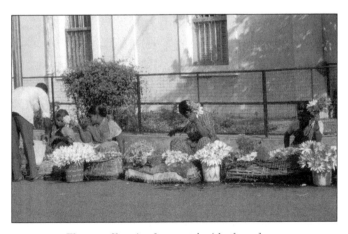

Flower sellers in the street beside the ashram

After breakfast, Dr Basu collected me and we went to take darshan (sight or vision) of Sri Aurobindo's room. The doctor's wife bought two bundles of pink and white lotus flowers, and gave us two each. We left our shoes at the stands lining the road opposite, and walked around to see Sri Aurobindo's room and living quarters. We queued in line. Everywhere official devotees were seated, keeping us in order, moving us, guiding us, and stopping us going through the wrong door. In the room there were some hanging silks and huge vases of vibrant fresh flowers. Devotees in the queue with us appeared to be hugely affected by the energy there, prostrating themselves and kissing the place on a chair where the Mother's feet had once been. Some prostrated their body flat out in front of the chair. That evening I went to the School Playground with the doctor and his family, for another meditation in the darkness.

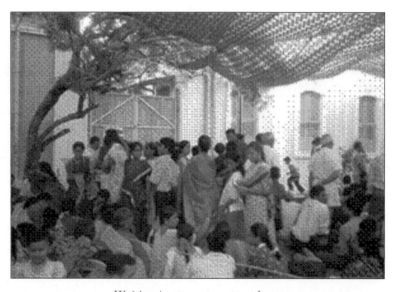

Waiting in queue to enter ashram

Special Meditation: Sri Aurobindo's body luminescence. Several days later on the morning of 9th December, there was another 6am meditation at the ashram. This was to commemorate the day Sri Aurobindo was interred. We were told Sri Aurobindo's body stayed luminous for five days after his death, and then on 9ᵗʰ December, the luminescence faded, and there was a meditation for remembrance on that day each year. Thousands of devotees gathered in Pondicherry. The *samadhi* became silently crowded in the cool pre-dawn air. I walked across the road to the comparative peace of the garden.

In the School Garden, I found a place to sit by the seventeen-petal Lotus flower fountain in the pond. I sat on the circular marble surround, underneath a tree with huge purple flowers that wove a circle of branches around the fountain and pond. It was still dark, bats were flying about, and there must have been several thousand people, settling themselves for the 6am meditation.

Public Meditations. My field trips to India coincided with several other anniversaries of Sri Aurobindo and the Mother, and I attended the group meditations at the ashram on these occasions. Thousands of people arrived in Pondicherry on such days from all over the country. Coach-loads travelled here for the meditation and *darshan*. The streets became crowded with vehicles and queues of followers waited to enter the sacred confines of the ashram.

After one New Year's mediation at 6am, huge queues formed in the streets, as up to 3,000 people took a flower or two and dropped some money in the box by the *samadhi*. This queuing continued for hours, and well into the afternoon. People bought flowers from the chattering flower sellers on the street corner. They queued in the street, around corners, carrying their flowers and money for the collection box. They queued right up to the sea front, then on arrival at the ashram, they filed past the *samadhi* in silence.

On Mother's Birthday (21st February) entry for *darshan* started even earlier, at 4am for emergency and essential workers. Some people slept all night in the queue. At 5.00 am, three streets were covered with tarpaulin, and coloured cloth sun shades stretched over ropes. By 5.30 am schoolchildren sat in neat rows ready to enter the ashram rooms. Thousands of people came into town, to visit the Mother's and Sri Aurobindo's room. By mid morning, the streets were crammed with parked cars, buses, coaches and cycles.

Later in the day, visitors queued for meal tickets at the Central Bureau so they could eat at the ashram Dining Hall. Officials guided people into cordoned areas with stringed-off pens. Thousands sat in string pens in the street for between 4 and 6 hours, waiting to go inside the ashram. In the street beyond there was a huge water tank, from which ashramites filled bottles of water with a small plastic mug and walked up and down the pens, inviting people to drink.

That evening when the streets became empty, they were littered with newspapers and water bottles, unusual for this town, which was normally so clean in the former French Quarter of Pondicherry.

Weight of philosophy. Sometimes I felt as if people had deified the Mother and Sri Aurobindo, but if they had, Dr Mistry said it was OK, for every time they honoured them, they tuned into the energy force those two humans brought down to earth. It seemed to me as if the gurus had been 'hindu-ised'. Some days I felt trapped by the weight of discipline and rituals. I thought that what had been and still was a major existential philosophy of life and cosmos, had somehow become a ritualised discipline. Occasionally I felt certain words taken to be sacred in Pondicherry, were judgemental, were related to a specific period in time, and sometimes belittled human beings and their troubles.

The words were beginning to affect me. I felt some were lacking in compassion, pursuing an ideal, and not acknowledging or accepting a person as they were. At that time I felt as if I was an imperfect being: I knew I suffered from melancholy and experienced mood swings, but hoped I honoured myself as I was, even as I aspired to be serene. I felt pressurised, as if I was expected to change, to conform to a norm. I felt frustrated with the attitude that illness must be overcome, and one could not achieve anything unless in good mental health.

On days when I felt disturbed, I sat in my room in Golconde and watched the reflection of water on the concrete slabs and on the ceiling. A reflection of wind, water and sun, and the very tranquillity of it seemed to calm me. I watched those patterns of sunlight on the white wall in my room, and wondered whether I would see those shadows when I was in spirit form. I was concerned my tears might be remembered by my soul and brought into a subsequent life for 'reworking'. At 3.30pm, I went downstairs to the garden in Golconde and sat with other residents, sipping tea and munching biscuits.

SUMMARY

This part of the research resulted in my visiting temples, a cathedral and two ashrams renowned for providing mental peace to those pilgrims who visited them. I had been anointed by water from the wells at Rameshwaram, and watched pilgrims conduct prayers for their dead on the shores of the Bay of Bengal. With colleagues I'd undertaken healing rituals at Vaitheeswarankoil, washed my feet in waters of the sacred tank, and heard about ancient libraries of palm leaf oracles. I had visited the museum of votive offerings beside the white cathedral to Our Lady at Vailankanni, and seen the thousands of items given in thanks for prayers answered

In search of strategies for mental peace, I'd visited temples dedicated to propitiating the planets like Suryanarkoil. I'd also stayed at two ashrams, Sri Ramana Maharshi and the Sri Aurobindo ashram in Pondicherry. As for my personal mental peace, sometimes it eluded me, sometimes it visited me, and I continued to aspire towards it.

In the following section, I explore cultural explanatory models for mental distress, looking at both mundane and esoteric theories of illness causation. I explore mundane triggers of distress like substance abuse or personal psychological problems, and I report on more esoteric beliefs, such as the role of planets, or past lives.

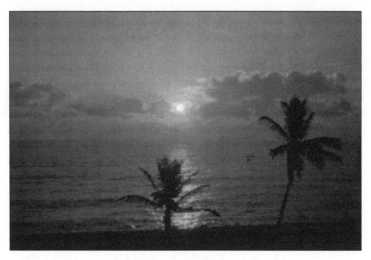

Sunrise in Pondicherry

PART THREE

EXPLANATORY MODELS FOR MENTAL DISTRESS

OVERVIEW OF PART THREE

Explanatory Models for Mental Distress

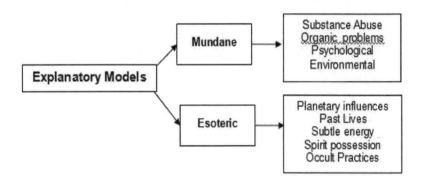

The treatment strategies suggested by practitioners and accepted by patients were directly influenced by their explanatory models for illness and their theories of illness causation. The diagnosis a psychiatrist made was based on a fusion of western psychiatric training, and his or her understanding of Indian frameworks of knowledge. The treatment accepted by the patient, was based on their respect for the doctor, and how well the diagnosis was accepted and fitted within their frameworks of knowledge and beliefs. From an analysis of interviews, there was a multiplicity of theories for illness causation, not only among patients but also among different kinds of practitioners. The fact that I interviewed people in a doctor's clinic may have skewed the responses I was given. In this section, I consider which explanatory models for mental distress held currency.

There were certain differences between factors psychiatrists and traditional healers believed caused mental distress and those influences their patient's mentioned. The mundane factors that triggered mental distress and malfunction were the most obvious and usually the first mentioned by patients. There were certain influences to mental disorder that occurred regardless of a person's sex, or marital state. However, as mentioned in chapter 4, there were certain influences that appeared to be specific to married or single women or men in India. In this chapter I set out mundane theories of causation of mental distress. This is followed by a chapter on esoteric explanations, including the role of spirit possession as a theory of causation.

The key causal factors mentioned by practitioners, psychiatrists, healers, or astrologers, are set out in chart 8.1 on the following page. Each topic is covered more fully in chapters 8 and 9 on mundane and esoteric explanatory models, in which I present both lay and professional perspectives in more detail.

CHART NO. 8.1
CAUSAL FACTORS WHICH INFLUENCE MENTAL DISORDER
(according to practitioners: psychiatrists & astrologers)

- **BIOLOGICAL:**
  - ○ Organic Disorders, Substance abuse

- **PSYCHOLOGICAL RESPONSES**
  - ○ Relational, social, political, economic
  - ○ Having desires or attachments, over-joy

- **DISEQUILIBRIUM**
  - ○ Disharmony between body, emotions and mind. Mismatch leading to disequilibrium, then disease
  - ○ Poor architecture or environmental surroundings
  - ○ Anger or non-propitiation of deities
  - ○ Curses

- **LOSS AND GENERATIONAL FACTORS**
  - ○ Loss of land, bereavement
  - ○ Misdeeds of relatives (current or deceased)
  - ○ Hereditary, inherited from ancestors

- **PLANETARY INFLUENCES & KARMA**
  - ○ Planetary alignments, current & at birth
  - ○ Karma: misdeeds in a previous life

- **SPIRIT POSSESSION**
  - ○ Problems with disembodied beings
  - ○ Occult 'forces' or energies

Chapter Eight

MUNDANE MODELS

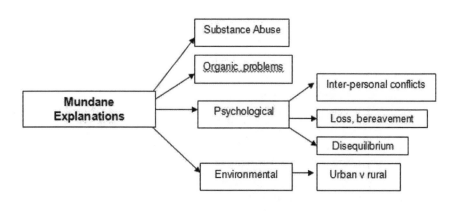

Mundane Factors affecting mental well being

The following mundane factors are considered to influence a person's well being and mental health:

- Substance abuse
- Physiological disorders
- Psychological responses
- Environmental factors
- Disequilibrium

Substance Abuse

Substance abuse was believed to be a common influence on mental health, whether alcohol, cannabis, heroin or others. I asked Dr Basu how he could tell the difference between young men in the locked nursing home who were heroin addicts, synthetic opiate addicts, or who had schizophrenia. I was told that each of the drugs had different withdrawal symptoms, so doctors could tell what had been taken. Schizophrenia had no withdrawal symptoms. Then he told me about the case of Ariram: when he came off the correct medication his thinking became illogical, whereas usually he was calm and an immaculately well spoken, educated, articulate young man.

Physiological disorders

Lay people differentiated organic brain disorder, due to tumour, accident, or malformation at birth, from functional disorder. Biological conditions were thought to be alleviated through the medium of prayer, but it was not considered appropriate for people in this situation to be restrained or housed at religious establishments. For example at the temple in Tiruvidaimarudur (mentioned in Chapter 6) there was one young man with Downs Syndrome, who used to follow the other men on their sacred perambulations around the temple, but unlike his companions, he was never restrained: he was free.

In Pondicherry, one of Dr Basu's neighbours had a brain tumour, and he used prayer to alleviate his symptoms. A devotee of Sri Aurobindo, once he could no longer work in his normal office job, the ashram employed him in the kitchens. Each morning he went to breakfast, collected a few white flowers from the tree beside the eating area. He walked flat-footed, his arms shaking like jelly, his hands held out in front. He spoke good English, and he said it was by the Mother's grace he was this well in spite of the tumour. Dr Basu said he managed to keep balance on his bike, through the power of prayer alone. He rode to the ashram every day, put the flowers on the *samadhi* and said a prayer.

Psychological responses

Psychological responses to poor relationships with family, neighbours, and colleagues could result in distress so severe as to warrant a visit to the psychiatrist. In particular married women who attended Dr Basu's clinics in Kolkata were there due to negative outcomes of patrilocal marriage, that is, after their wedding they went to live with their husband's family, and became that family's responsibility. Being the last to come into the family, those not treated well were used as domestic servants and labourers. If their husband's brothers later married, then the situation might ease as they received domestic help from their incoming sisters in law. Another cause of mental distress leading to disorder was if they failed to conceive a child, or had one late after years of marriage. Sometimes distress was due to post natal depression, or fatigue from doing domestic work too soon after their child's birth. For single girls over 20, the strain was sometimes caused through being of unmarried status.

Severe distress could also be caused by economic problems and perceived political injustices. However, one man's mental disorder was caused by joy. He was a taxi driver (no.11 HS) belonging to the schedule cast, who trained himself to become a lawyer. His brother drove the cab in the morning and he drove it from 2 to 9 pm. He used to study in the morning and when he had completed his law degree (LLB), he had a mental breakdown through happiness. He was overjoyed, then burnt out, came to Dr Basu's notice, and stayed in the locked nursing home. He described himself as a peasant who became a solicitor. Once recovered, he was an advocate in the law courts. He planned to go back to his village to practise law.

There were several students I interviewed: one had pressure of work and problems with a girlfriend. The other was concerned about human abuses to the environment, and he distrusted previous medical interventions offered to him. The third was a young female student who distrusted her father's actions.

Loss and mental distress. Loss could be either loss of a relationship, death and bereavement, loss of one's native place, separation from one's land, being a refugee, or having political or economic hardship. A number of patients were refugees who had moved from Bangladesh to Kolkata looking for a better life, fleeing from harsh conditions there. Several times Dr Basu mentioned patients who were refugees from Bangladesh had problems settling in Kolkata. They were experiencing loss of their land and relationship patterns in one area.

The psychiatrist Eisenbruch[54] conducted research with refugees and displaced peoples into the effect of external life events on mental health such as migration and loss of land. He expanded the theme of collective grief in relation to loss of a homeland, whereby loss of the perception of self occurs together with massive life changes. One of Dr Basu's cousins noted: *"Housing has to be suitable to avoid mental distress. There is a particular problem with refugees, who are removed from the environment they know, from their own homes, their own way of life, and those with whom they had social bonds, and their childhood memories. When the outer envelope is changed too much, then there may be psychiatric problem: social disorder and personal breakdown occur."*

Loss and death. There were several other instances cited as possible triggers for loss of self and going off balance: one was when patients had seen an unnatural death earlier in their life, and this had affected their mind and behaviour. This factor was mentioned in general as a trigger for a number of patients of either sex, whether single or married. For example, the gentle unmarried woman of thirty (KM) who kept trying to hang herself: apparently when she was a child, about six years old, she had seen someone hang themselves in front of her. The man in the Nursing home (RP) who also repeatedly tried to hang himself, was aware that two of his father's sisters' sons had committed suicide. The woman (SR) who walked on railway lines at night trying to kill herself, in spite of having a very supportive husband, had become frightened after seeing a murder as a child. Also one of her close friends had died in a cycle accident around that time. There were patterns of repeated deaths in her family, with her father and his brother having died on the same date, one year apart.

This type of pattern of events had been reported in Europe by Canault[55]. She gave examples of French psychologists who claimed an individual may experience trans-generational sickness, whereby hidden grief or unresolved trauma was suppressed but surfaced in the memory or behaviour of subsequent generations. It was passed on until it was revealed or resolved. Psychologists suggested suppression may result in psychosis in later generations. She said in such cases, becoming conscious of the secret promoted healing and enhanced mental health. People also believed well-being could be influenced by generational factors such as the misdemeanours of current or deceased relatives, or by hereditary factors that continued through the ancestral bloodline. Thus it was not only personal misdeeds, which could affect a person's health.

Environmental Factors

The balance of mental health could be influenced by environmental factors such as poor domestic or community architecture. Practitioners were aware of a set of architectural *shastras*, or ancient Hindu treatises, which gave directions on how a house should be built, its design and layout. In practice, such suggestions were only followed by those familiar with them, who could afford them. Occupants of dwellings who had mental problems did from time to time seek the advice of a specialist practitioner. A *vastusilpi*, or traditional architect, sensed a person's situation from the energy vibrations of their house, and suggested alternative healing designs. A skilled practitioner would see from the foundations alone that inhabitants had social or health problems. Practitioners offered suggestions for rectifying designs that caused unhappiness or unease in a property.

He explained architectural specialists (*vastusilpi*) were aware of subtle energy and this influenced the way they designed buildings. He reminded us that rules created for human benefit in one part of India, would not be suitable in another geographical area. For example "*in an area designed to allow in the cool winds in the south, the same design used in the northern states, would give people a chill. In areas where they have severe weather conditions, if they follow the rules of the Chinese Feng Shui, or the Hindu vastas (architectural specialist) it would be utterly inappropriate.*"

He talked about the problems of ready-made environments, the changing requirements of the family, and the frustrations of living in a ready-made home. *"Entire cities are designed on paper, with unsuitable living spaces, of unsuitable size, and unsuitable communal areas. I think human beings are the last to be considered in city designs. We have developed settlement out of economic need. We have adopted technology without thinking about it. People are living inside pipes, you can see them in Kolkata. People have been under severe strain and pressure by the technology and economics, which have neglected humans. We need to find some order."*

Environment factors and Healing. The medical herbalist Loganathan mentioned environmental factors and their effect on healing. His forefathers had practised herbal medicine for eleven generations. When he was a child, he remembered meeting his grandfather who was very old, and hearing how he treated mental health patients. His grandfather, who specialised in addressing mental distress, said energies of land and geographical space could affect a person's mental health. Illness might not only be from the land, but might also occur from friction between relatives who lived in close proximity. He wasn't sure which strategy resulted in cure: being looked after by relatives, prayers at the temple, or being removed from a location of tension.

If a patient came to his grandfather with a problem due to place, he would ask if they had relatives in distant settlements, then he would suggest they stay with those relatives to reduce negative influences. He would advise the relatives how to look after the patient correctly and to feed him or her well. He would instruct them how to make a prayer with the relevant herbs, then offer them to the relevant deity, but not to the patient (unless specified). They would do this for 30 days, in order to effect a cure. This would allow heated situations time to cool down. *"Mental disorder is due to different factors. For example mental illness* in the village regions is entirely different from mental patients in the city areas. When it occurs in the city areas, it is due to drug abuse, alcohol abuse, financial reasons, and family separations. These are the main problems we see when patients from the towns. When patients come from the villages it is mainly for social problems." There was also a belief that the architecture, compound walls, type of roof, room size and location could disturb mental peace, and the following kinds of treatment strategies were undertaken to address this and remedy the environment.

He mentioned a specific kind of architecture that would help people with mental disorders. "*There is one traditional system called vastu. This system means for each person's horoscope a specific number of feet are required to construct a house, any building, even a marriage hall. So we have to follow the correct calculations, and inside the building we have to follow the different elements, kitchen, bathroom and toilet. Also outside we have to pay attention. This is based on the nakshetra, the stars of the horoscope. We have to work out the directions of the east, west, north and south, and in the inner circle we should see what plants need to be maintained, the size of the rooms and the location and positioning of the different objects in each room. All this is based on the stars, the stars responsible for this particular horoscope. It all needs to be worked out as part of vastu.*"

However, Dr Basu's cousin Gautam reminded us: "*people here only have 30 by 60 plots of land. They cannot do much in the vastu system. The streets are narrow and we have to build houses in this or that direction. Vastu specialists cannot follow those who live in the city. However, inside the home one can make alterations, and this is helpful in giving peace to the mind. Through colours we can find out the best one for peace of mind.*"

Urban and Rural Responses. Dr Basu explained about the different ways people responded in urban and rural environments: "*The perception of what is well is different in different places. In our rural society, they are adjusted. The chronic cases would just roam around the* *field or around the village taking food. Whereas in the city there are problems, if you don't go to work you are a burden on your relatives.*

"For example, these wandering sadhus, there are groups of these wandering holy men all over India. There are a considerable number of them who suffer from simple schizophrenia. You will always find this among wandering sadhus. It suited their life-style, they go from place to place, having no food and begging. Nowadays it doesn't suit so many, so they go around picking up food from the dustbins."

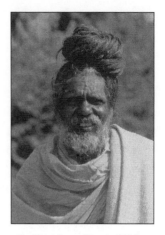

Sadhu, Jean Pierre Ribière

"Secondly in our rural areas, men roam in the fields. Otherwise they are not causing any nuisance. They are just wandering about, talking to themselves, coming and getting food and going out. The family income is derived from the paddy, which is growing in the fields, and nobody considers the men to be a burden. It is only in our modern society where we have compartmentalised, and where we live in small rooms, that they are out of place."

"How do we assess who is well, who is not disturbing? In older times patients were coming to our clinic. We used to tell them it is not always possible to have a clinical recovery, but a social recovery is possible. By social recovery I mean they can take their own food, take a bath, go for a walk. If they can do that normally then they will not disturb others. A social recovery is acceptable. One who is not fully clinically recovered, but is still relating within society, his quality of life is better."

"The quality of life of a patient who is in a rural area, in a village, who has not fully recovered clinically, but has some amount of social recovery, his quality of life may be better than a person in a city with the same illness who has more clinical recovery."

"Does that mean that the definition of mental illness can change according to location?" *"Yes, yes and it is so much linked to the environment. It is linked to what we call culture. It depends how much we can accept, and what our level of tolerance is."*

He mentioned some people considered mentally ill were taken to healing places, like temples and shrines, and left by their relatives, who never returned to collect them. *"This is practised everywhere even in our mental nursing homes. There is an advance fee of one month even if they only stay for five days. They give a false address. All mental hospitals and private nursing clinics, they have four or five patients like that, who have never been taken home. This is a common problem everywhere."*

Dr Basu explained people with similar symptoms may have quite different experiences depending on whether they lived in a rural or an urban environment. He told us about the differences between social recovery and clinical recovery, and what it meant for a person's quality of life. He mentioned those who had been taken for health care treatments, and then abandoned by their families. This seemed as if stigma and discrimination might be culturally determined, and based on environmental surroundings.

Disequilibrium

I interviewed practitioners who were devotees of Sri Aurobindo, about their beliefs and explanations for mental ill health. They considered when there was a lack of harmony between a person's body, emotions and mind, the mismatch would result in disequilibrium, and then disease. I also heard discussions about imbalance being caused by deities which were angry or undertook mischievous activities if they felt they were not being adequately propitiated. Some practitioners considered planetary alignment at birth would affect a person's well being, as could karmic effects (one's own misdemeanours in previous lives), generational influences, and the effects of the unquiet dead. People claimed disharmony could also be caused if a person had desires or attachments to material things or relationships, and these would result in mental distress.

Dr Alok Pandey the psychiatrist I spoke to in Pondicherry, informed me that "*two different illnesses can arise from the same psychological source. The Mother mentions illness is disequilibrium of the inner being, so the same disequilibrium in the inner level, can lead to two very different diseases*".

"*Perhaps at a physical level it is easier to understand, for example if my liver, my heart and kidneys are not in harmony with each other, there is no proper exchange of information, or they are disjointed from each other, this is liable to cause illness. We go to the psychological roots and you can help the patient change their attitude and thereby initiate the healing process from within, outwards.*"

He continued: *Similarly in our inner being, all of these organs are symbolic of a deeper psychological truth. Let us say we have a lower vital nature, as in Sri Aurobindo's taxonomy of consciousness, we have a higher vital nature and a mental nature. All of these parts may not work in harmony. A man may have beautiful ideas, but the lower vital may be stuck with greed. This will cause disharmony. If the mind and lower vital are going together, even at a lower level, a person is relatively free, but if one part is progressing and the other is not progressing, it causes disruption, and that inner fracture is revealed outwardly as illness. So the whole view will change.*"

I asked Dr Basu to set out his view about how illness manifests in the body. *"We see how the different planes of consciousness have manifested one after the other in evolution until the mind has been reached. Yet Sri Aurobindo says that the human being is not a finished product, like in a sense, a flower is a finished product. It is so specific, so beautiful, you can tell it is something really complete in its totality. But humans feel that they are imperfect, that they have to develop. They don't feel as if they have developed all their potentialities to the maximum extent. They have that yearning to grow more and more. From a consciousness perspective, you can see how the planes have manifested one after another: the plane of matter that is represented by the physical body, the plane of life energy, and the plane of mind have sequentially evolved."*

He explained about harmony required for the different levels of awareness, and how illness might occur. *"We see that the complete harmonising of all the planes have not yet occurred in a human being. Consider that our physical body, our emotions and our mind are not properly harmonised. The mind might want something that our body might not want. Our emotions might want something that our mind doesn't want. The mismatching which goes on results in dis-equilibrium, and that can lead to a disease. A better harmonisation of the different planes of our being can be facilitated when we shift the centre of integration from the ego to a 'beyond-ego' principle. This shift is necessary for a holistic development of our being and is a harbinger of integral health."*

Dr Basu claimed disharmony between the different planes of consciousness manifested on the physical plane as ill health, and suggested if we could address inner disharmony, then we could effect healing. In his book[56] he explained the planes of consciousness at which various therapies worked including pharmacological drugs, acupuncture, energy healing, and psychotherapy. He defined the characteristics of the different planes of consciousness and ended each chapter with ideas for research, in order to explore an integral health programme. He suggested with regard to health-seeking strategies, instead of searching from therapy to therapy, we should focus on how they each relate to the different planes of consciousness.

He explained why people who engaged in spiritual practices might fall ill. *"Even seekers who are not concentrating on the outer personality but decide to become very spiritual do not automatically qualify for holistic health. They might develop their inner being in such a way, that the outer being is neglected. So again there is a mismatch between the inner being and the outer being. That is the reason you will find that many people who practice occultism and spirituality fall ill, because certain parts of their being are more developed than others. So the mismatch is between different levels, different perspectives. We are not perfect. The more we learn to harmonise the different parts of our personality, the more we learn to harmonise the different planes of our consciousness, the more we can rise above ill health, we can rise above disease."*

❖ ❖ ❖

SUMMARY

After interviewing practitioners at Sri Aurobindo ashram, I learnt mundane factors influencing mental well being included: organic problems like brain tumours; substance abuse from alcohol or heroin; and psychological problems due to inter-personal conflicts or loss of a loved one. I was also made aware responses to mental ill health might be quite different depending on whether a person lived in an urban or rural environment. There were also concerns about balance and harmony and the psychiatrists interviewed here stressed the importance of looking after the mind, body and spirit together.

Chapter Nine

ESOTERIC
MODELS

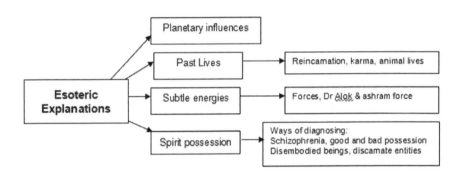

Introduction: Lay perspectives on mental health

Lay people had different beliefs on the triggers of mental ill-health. These included a 'spiritual force' that was too strong for visitors to the Sri Aurobindo ashram to contain, and children who were born with learning difficulties after being animals in previous lives. I discovered the latter after visiting a home for special needs girls on the outskirts of Pondicherry (Jwala Home for Mental Peace). Another perspective was obtained after talking to an astrologer / clairvoyant, and a third from a discussion with a medical herbalist. Some lay people had a mechanical or plumbing perception of the brain, and felt there was 'something loose' if a person experienced mental distress.

Esoteric factors considered to influence a person's well being and mental health by both lay people and professional practitioners included:

- Planetary influences
- Past lives and reincarnation
- Subtle influences
- Spirit possession

Planetary influences on mental health.

Many people considered it important to honour and propitiate the planets, and believed this was essential for their mental well being. In Pondicherry, Dr Loganathan, the medical herbalist, claimed there were various planetary influences, which both caused mental illness and facilitated various treatments. The effects of the planets on a person's mind could be neutralised by plants and herbal medicine. He had written a book in Tamil, correlating plants with planets and the elements. He said plant remedies a traditional herbalist prepared, depended under what planet their client was born. Specific plants came under the influence of different planets. Both patients and plants were influenced by planetary alignments.

Loganathan explained how by using calculations based on a patient's birth chart he would determine the good and bad periods in a patient's life. Using the horoscope a practitioner would assess which herbal medicine should be given, from which part of the plant, at a particular astrological time. "*By going in deep to calculate the degrees of the elevation of the planet, and linking that with their lifetime, one can note that this time, this particular planet has a major role influencing this person. We can determine what the peak period is of this planet, for this person. For this period, if the planet is not in a good position of the person's chart, it may reflect in their behaviour, or it may lead to an improvement of the disease."*

"There are planets responsible for health and education, and family. Each planet has different responsibilities, according to its combination with others. One has to see the degree of elevation of each planet to see whether they cause mental illness. Alternatively mental ill health could be due to other members of the family, which must be taken into consideration. If we don't look at all of this, we may misunderstand the horoscope, and the plant selected for treatment may not be the most helpful."

The ancient practitioners used to define the cause of mental illness according to planetary influences, and then explored which plant was correct for treatment. *"Once you have worked out the real cause of mental health, then we can look at what plant can be used to alleviate the effect of this planet. For example in the case of the moon, worshipping the correct plant and giving medicine from it would lead to a reduction of the symptoms."*

Practitioners used to consult ancient literary sources, the yoga sutra, which outlined all the problems of mental illness due to hereditary effects. Loganathan explained: *"this means the different karmas, and the different actions performed, not by the patient, but the patient's father or forefathers, lead to this problem in this generation. Once the karma stops, so the next generation of that family will be normal."*

Past Lives, Karma, and Mental Ill Health

Dr Loganathan believed past lives could affect a person's mental health. He suggested for some patients the effect of karma and the planets may not be cleared in one lifetime. The planetary period may last for over 20 years, and during this time a patient may die. *"We also suggest this is due to the karma of the generation of their forefather's, and it is linked to their life now. So please understand that this is the life and they are suffering, and with them, this karma may end, or it may not. We do not know."*

"One can also see that by looking at the horoscope, whether the karma will end with this, or whether the karma will be left to the next generation. In that case you have to see the horoscope of the next generation to see when it will end."

"Karma means action: frightening somebody, or misusing some ones' property, or taking somebody's property, money or material things. These planetary laws may be different from those followed by the government or the administration. The patient may be considered a punishable man by the government, but by the horoscope he may look very normal. We need to consider everything: the land, the karma, his life-style, and the type of living he performs. All these things play an important role in mental illness."

Earlier I had asked him whether someone's past lives could affect their mental health. In fact the answer he gave me indicated that the situation was far more complex than I had begun to understand. *"We are looking at another dimension. The exchange of the genetic material in the crossover of the chromosomes, that factor is unique. And the type of genetic material transferred, and the type of precognition occurs during that time. This is due to the action of the forefather's, and the influence of the planets, and the planets' movements. It is not just the movement of planets, but the planets themselves actually influence the good and bad moments of the person and their behaviour in life."*

Past Lives and Learning Difficulties. I was taken to visit the Jwala Home for Mental Peace on the outskirts of Pondicherry on the road towards Cuddalore. An elderly woman from a wealthy family had established it in the mid 1990's, after she lost her grown-up son in an accident, and decided to devote herself to charity. She had worked as a psychiatric nurse, and when she set up this home, she selected those girls with learning difficulties who were calm, so none would disturb any of the others.

A younger woman in her 30's helped look after the children. This small hostel stood alone, with its headboard indicating its reason for existence: Jwala Home for Mental Peace. On the day I went to visit, 12 girls aged from 4 to 15 were seated on the mat in front of us. Some girls sat quietly, others grinned to themselves. One had spontaneous uncontrollable movements of her body and hands. They all seemed in harmony with each other and got on well. The girls were well dressed and well fed with their hair brushed.

However, there was just one problem: Dr Basu said three girls were mentally normal. They sat on the floor with all the others who had 'congenital organic mental retardation'. Each of them had been rejected by their families. One was a four year old deaf mute, with a 'lazy' arm. She could do all the children's puzzles she was given and had clear eyes and good inter-relationships. Another was a 14 year old girl, whose mother had schizophrenia, didn't recognise her and had rejected her. She had studied in school, had some English, but was depressed. The third girl was there because her parents had both died, and her brother had rejected her. She was bright eyed and articulate.

The psychiatrist felt the normal girls should be trained to assist as helpers, by looking after the others, so they could learn to cook and gain some self-respect. The youngest child should be sent to school. His concern was nobody would take them in marriage, and they might become outcaste.

In order to be taken into this home, the girls had to be certified as 'mentally retarded'. The medical superintendent had put their IQ at a low level. Recently the government offered the owner 250 rupees a month for each girl, but none of it had been paid. The psychiatrist felt the home should establish a policy, which stated how the girls were accepted there, with clear criteria for entry, how they should be trained and educated when they were there, how they might be encouraged to leave, and where they should go when they were sixteen. He felt there were funds the school could target from the government and the state: it was curious that only one girl there attracted state funding, 250 rupees a month, while the director was always struggling for food.

The man who brought us was an ashramite and he carried a gift of a cassette player for the children. He wanted to play the Mother's organ music for the girls. He suggested the owner play the music in the mornings and evening, since it would be of great benefit to the girls. He believed it would lift the girls' souls to a new level of consciousness, heal their brains, and release them from handicap.

Mental health, reincarnation and rebirth. There was an explanation for those children who were born with what local people called "mental retardation". An American pilgrim in Pondicherry told me about her belief that all mentally retarded children were actually former animals, incarnating for the first time and not yet ready to be fully human. Later I heard a similar belief again: that any form of mental handicap was because the person was incarnating as a human being for the first time. Although this was some people's belief, others felt laws of rebirth and karma should not be mechanistically and simplistically interpreted.

Reincarnation beliefs were ubiquitous among Asians in India, and those who migrated to UK[57]. I did not know whether the stories I heard were myth or reality, but as they were certainly present in people's thoughts and in their narratives, they were the informant's realities: they were data. I was told stories by those who lived in Pondicherry and Auroville, both native Indian and resident foreigners.

Subtle Influences on Mental Health

The continuum between spiritual experience and mental health has been recognised in the west[58], and today, more people are considering the effects of subtle influences on mental well being[59]. In this section I present examples of Indian beliefs about subtle and occult influences on mental health.

In India the term occult did not carry the same baggage as in the west. It meant hidden, and was value laden in a different way. Dr Basu explained what he meant by the term 'occultist'. "*By occult I mean, something that is hidden, which can't be seen. There are forces in the cosmic consciousness which can be harnessed and manipulated when these practices have been done for years. They are there in the collective unconscious, and the collective psyche of mankind, and can be used and manipulated*".

He mentioned specialists in occult power, who cannot control the energies, and attend his clinics for psychiatric help: "*I have also seen these occult healers, these occultists themselves becoming psychiatric patients, becoming mad, because they can't control the power they develop. Even on occasion there were one or two I told them to stop the practice."* The key example of this was the man I interviewed SB, the clairvoyant astrologer, who shifted back and forwards from psychotic patient to practitioner.

The force at Pondicherry. There were more explanatory models for mental illness concerned with subtle energy. I had heard several stories and rumours that the strength of energy or 'force' around the *samadhi* in the Ashram could detrimentally influence a person's mental health. I was told the Mother used to send people away for rehabilitation to a distant place where the force of the *samadhi* energy could not affect them. They were sent to a mental nursing home, sedated with allopathic medicine, and then collected by their families. These narratives, whether true or false seemed embedded in stories around Pondicherry and Auroville.

To try and gain a bit of clarity, I asked Amitava, a colleague of the psychiatrist from Kolkata, whether people believed there was a particular force around the *Samadhi* in Pondicherry. I wanted to know what happened to people if the force was too strong for them. He replied: *"A mother cannot do any harm to her children. It is a powerful motherly force, but it doesn't hurt anyone. If someone pulls at it ambitiously and gets more energy than they can handle, then it is a problem. It can be troublesome. They may become mad. It is a high energy for them, so they may feel tired or ill. Or they can go astray with this power, if they think it is their own, and misuse it."*

I heard a similar story several times, about the force of energy around the ashram, and its influence on people who experienced mental health problems. I did not know whether there was one story repeated and retold in different guises, whether it was part of a myth, or if there were different actual incidents. Whichever it was, these tales were part of the 'story threads' of the place.

Those who meditated in the ashram repeatedly said there was a force of energy there. They report the Mother said the energy was too strong for babies and mentally ill people, and they shouldn't be in its vicinity. Later I heard discussions among the medical doctors: there was a suggestion that the modern residence and centre being considered for the mentally distressed should be built a little distant from Pondicherry, so vibrations from the *samadhi* complex would not be too strong and adversely affect the patients within.

Subtle Triggers for Mental Distress. There were several narratives about subtle triggers for mental distress. In order to throw light on this, I had a chat with Dr Alok Pandey, the psychiatrist then working as Wing Commander with the Air Force in Bangalore. He mentioned a multiplicity of triggers that might result in mental distress: biological (brain patterns, chemical and genetic effects); social (bereavement, isolation, sudden loss events); and psychological triggers in personality, those identified by modern psychiatry. He expressed the concern that medical students and some psychiatrists got carried away by 'material and mechanistic' aspects of life and health.

He believed a person's psychic consciousness and spiritual personality should also be included in assessment. If a person's spiritual side was developed, if there was a spiritual element, he felt people could go through life protected against mental distress, even in difficult circumstances. He thought it ideal that a person should also have 'solid nerves' or a solid base (*nadha*: nature). Without 'solid nerves' a person may experience:*"information overload: they may vibrate to every kind of force, and the chances of having a breakdown are much more….. It is through the nerves that we come into contact with the world and the forces around."*

Dr Pandey also mentioned subtle forces of a psychological nature, which could influence a human being. These included feelings of anger or jealousy that could be exchanged between people, and those collective ones we might pick up from a crowd in a bar or pub. *"When we go to a place of worship, or a graveyard, the atmospheres are different. In a mob or crowd, a person's general consciousness comes down. Collective psychology overrides individual psychology, unless the person is a very developed being".*

"There are always psychological forces, which affect us, for example, anger in one person can induce anger in another. We can get caught up in it, and keep on inter-changing our psychological atmosphere with others. Occultists would call this 'subtle energy'. Such people may see a wave or a vibration. I don't know, I don't see such things. But what all of us experience, is that psychological forces affect us, and we also pour out, like receivers and transmitters, a number of psychological forces, which emanate and effect people".

I was wondering if this might include empathy, with which a practitioner can tune into their patient, or mindfulness. He said: *"our patients can be affected by the psychological atmosphere in which they live. Equally they can get healed if their psychiatrist emanates a very peaceful vibration within himself. So it works both ways."*

He had heard there might be certain forces around graveyards, though he didn't experience them himself. He felt prayers held there helped to contain any such 'forces'. He thought certain types of people might *"attract some disembodied being who may occupy such places. These disembodied beings are more likely to be present at the site of accidents, or violent crimes. Whereas in the graveyard there are very often prayers, so they may be contained, and move on."*

However, he continued *"I have experience of patients who attended to people who died a violent death, suicide, or similar things. And that was the first point where they had a neurotic break down, or panic attacks, which continued for 5 or 6 years. I had patients like that. So I guess to some extent environmental consciousness and disembodied beings can influence patients, if they are receptive. But, there are so many people who are not receptive."* The topic of disembodied beings and spirit possession frequently came up in narratives. In order to expand my understanding I continued to ask practitioners about it.

Spirit Possession and Mental Health

Sometimes Dr Basu intuitively felt one of his clients developed mental disorder as a result of being possessed, whereas at other times he took advice about causation from traditional healers and occultists. Some of his clients had explanatory models that involved influence by occult or non-physical entities. For example one female patient arrived at Dr Basu's home, out of working hours, with her family. They were of the opinion that she'd had black magic placed on her in the past, and needed the psychiatrist's assistance to dissolve the effects. Interesting people felt his clinic or presence could address occult effects. He was also open to the possibility a patient's previous life impinged on their present, or that they might be overshadowed or possessed by the spirit of a dead person.

During my stay informants gave me a lot of material on spirit possession and subtle influences as explanatory models for mental health. The information below comes from interviews with: the psychiatrists Drs Basu and Pandey, the Muslim cleric al Haji Saheb, a homoeopathic physician, and a couple of lay people with interest in such things. I wanted to know how they thought a discarnate being might be created, and how they told the difference between a person needing psychiatric help and one requiring help from different healers.

How are disembodies being created? Dr Pandey explained the way he thought disembodied beings were created, and how they could overshadow and influence a living person. He explained disembodied beings exist in the vital world, the world of vitality and emotions, that few people except for specialists (like psychics or mediums) can observe directly. He told me that most of us don't have the skills and sensitivity to see these worlds: *"Maybe this ignorance is a grace. If we were very aware of these things, it would make life very difficult. We cannot even handle the physical beings we are in contact with. It is a grace that we are not aware of others. It protects us and shields us. Because of this they come and pass, and are not able to induce any fear in most of us."*

Dr Pandey suggested they may be created by their being thrown out suddenly at death from their bodies, during which time some bystanders might catch them, like a spirit possession or attachment. He explained his understanding of the mechanism: *"our body is like a receptacle, a container, or a vessel, which contains many forces. It is like a receiver and a transmitter, like the TV, which crosses many different levels of vibration. Depending on what we are tuned to, we receive one force, which may or may not be revealed to others. Disembodied beings occur when the body disintegrates. Then these beings become disembodied, and they float freely in the environment, from where some people can catch them. Not everyone can catch them".*

He continued and explained to me how this influenced mental health, and he identified problems that resulted when practitioners used drugs alone to combat symptoms: *"Sri Aurobindo puts it very clearly, speaking of insanity, which can be a case of possession. Insanity can be due to possession by these disembodied beings, these hostile beings. Hysteria is nothing other than pressure from the vital world. Epileptic seizures can result from resistance to attack from these vital worlds. So there are these entities that are of a different substance and energy combination from us physical beings."* He informed me once an entity became attached to a human being, they may have trouble reincarnating, and get stuck on the earth's plane after they die. *"Yes, it is very difficult for some to be reborn. They are using many lower vital forces or real vital beings, who can make them do anything they want."* [Definition: A vital being may hold semi-conscious sensations, urges and desires, and expresses itself through emotions.]

A colleague joined our conversation and said he had experienced subtle beings. Mr Sircar had been an air traffic controller for the first 20 years of his career, had worked abroad, and retired from Chennai as the director of Commercial and Air-force Services. He lived in Pondicherry, and was very interested in Sri Aurobindo's philosophy of life. During his lifetime he had experiences, which went beyond the five senses. In his youth he met a man who had the special skills of deliberately possessing spirits to invite them to work as healers. *"He had control of some beings under him. In Bengali it is called 'pishar sidha', that is this gentleman could possess spirits: those entities were under his control. He used those entities for curing people; he used to give medicine. That man invoked the spirits and asked them to bless water, which was then given to the patients."* This sounded like skills of practicing shamans elsewhere in the world.

Mr Sircar claimed he discovered for himself the curative powers of prayer, whether uttered in English or Bengali. He believed that prayer helped relieve suffering, not only of living people, but discarnate entities who were caught on the earth's plane. He himself was not interested in contacting discarnate beings. I wondered whether he thought people who were in mental distress and seeing a psychiatrist, might actually be having experiences due to discarnate beings, but didn't know what was happening. *"I have come to believe, but I can't prove it, that mental aberrations in most cases are possession by other consciousnesses and other beings. People suddenly start behaving in a funny way. I believe they are possessed by some other forces. If someone is open to those forces, they can cause harm. A fellow student had a problem, and the doctors couldn't do anything, but when her family went to the oja (traditional healer), they found what happened and offered a remedy. I also know if people tell stories of ghosts, it can create thought formations."*

Good Possession. Amitava (a colleague of Dr Basu) told me about the concept of good possession, similar to that by Mr Sircar, whereby helpful spirits over-shadowed a person, allowed them enhanced clairvoyance, and gave them healing insights. *"Some people get possessed by good spirits, and many people who had illnesses or who are suffering, go to these possessed people. They have specific times when they are possessed, say once a week or twice a week. During their possessed state they say which medicine is required: you take this medicine or you take that medicine."*

"They have a special clarity when they are possessed. Hindus and Muslims all go to such people. Irrespective of religion, Hindus go to Muslims, Muslims to Hindus." This was something I had noticed before in India: no matter what one's birth religion, if a practitioner of another religious persuasion was renowned as powerful, then he or she attracted attention from all faiths. This also applied to powerful shrines or buildings that had a reputation for efficacy.

However, he said there was the concept of bad possession, where people were controlled by malevolent spirits. In Britain the research of psychiatrist Simon Dein attests to the relevance of this topic for UK residents[60]. I was confused between the symptoms of mental illness, spirit possession and those of schizophrenia. I was told the symptoms of spirit possession were similar to those of schizophrenia in the UK. However, the use of the term schizophrenia in India appeared to be different. I'd heard Dr Basu use the term 'simple schizophrenia', and so I asked him what it meant. *"Basically it means when one withdraws socially. Social withdrawal is the most important symptom. It is withdrawal from everybody. They don't socialise. They don't interact with other people. They remain alone, confined to themselves".*

Distinguishing Possession.

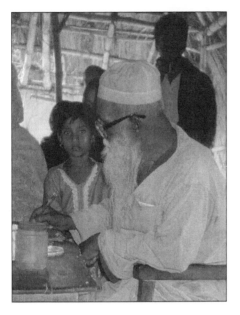

Muslim cleric's surgery

The Muslim cleric I met on the Bangladesh borders said he had a way of distinguishing between possession and psychiatric illness (see more extensive notes in Chapter 2). He himself dealt with those cases of spirit possession, through prayer and protective amulets, while those he considered had organic mental illness, he sent to the psychiatric clinic.

He explained how spirits were created: "*beings of another world have different types of bodies, or subtle bodies, and they can move in subtle ethereal space. Sometimes they come and have a bad influence on human beings, and that causes illness. These beings are of a different world, of a different dimension, which we usually cannot visualise and they can cause illnesses.*"

I wanted to know how he could distinguish possession and was told: "*Through practise he can visualise them, as an impression, like a silhouette. An act of illness may be manifested in the sort of attacks we see that give fits and fever, where the eyeballs roll up...*" One of his patients was Mohammad, a young man who he sent on to Dr Basu. He told me this man's elder sister had undergone a possession state by a *djinn*, but when he kept quarrelling with his sister, this upset the *djinn*, who didn't like him quarrelling with its 'client'. Thus he said her *djinn* triggered his psychiatric illness.

Physicians and possession. In the west a number of professionals have suggested there was some kind of similarity between spiritual experience and psychotic experience, that is, the symptoms were similar[61]. I wanted to understand more about physicians' perceptions of the perceived relationship between possession and mental illness, and so I talked to other doctors. I asked the senior homoeopathic physician at the clinic in Pondicherry if he had ever dealt with cases pertaining to be spirit possession. Dr Pachegaonkar had tackled and cured cases of schizophrenia and manic depression. These were diagnosed and treated by allopathic doctors, before being presented to him. He said there were examples where his homoeopathic treatment had averted a person's admission to psychiatric hospital. In such cases, he felt credit should go to the family because they provided good support for the sufferer. He explained about people who behaved strangely, heard voices, or apparently had discarnate spirits around them. I asked whether he ever had cases like that. *"Yes we have confronted such cases, where people believed that they were possessed by the spirits. Homoeopathically we look at such things. We have remedies for the condition whereby a person is easily magnetised, easily influenced by other beings. We call them easily magnetised. We take it as a symptom that a person is susceptible to such influences."*

I asked Dr Pachegaonkar, whether this formed part of his own belief system that there could be spirit entities: *"Earlier, we used to believe some spirits were there, but now we believe that even if such influences are there, for example if murder has occurred in one place, influences of the criminal mentality may remain for centuries. This I have read, but here and now we look at such things from a clinical angle, that the persons who are susceptible to it, alone would suffer from it, not everyone would be affected. The person who is not susceptible to it will not suffer from such influences."*

Dr Basu mentioned a case he dealt with the previous week in his surgery in Kolkata. *"I had a case last week where I also gave medicine. Last week I felt I had a case of spirit possession. A lady jumped in the pond last week, and she was brought to me. The pond was in front of her house, and that lady had a six month old child. My intuition was telling me strongly that this was a case of spirit possession. So I asked whether anyone else had ever had jumped into that pond."* He knew that post partum depression was a common thing, but they told him that other people had died in that pond. *"In east Bengal we have many ponds: one or two people will die, or they will commit suicide and die by drowning. So some kind of energy is there which attracts mishaps like these. So I felt that something like this was happening. I gave her medicines, and I said that if she didn't respond to them, I would also give an ECT, because I don't want to take any risks. Simply I told them to put camphor in the house (used by priests to purify the atmosphere)."*

Then there was the case of the unmarried woman KM (no.9 Chapter Two). When she was young, she had seen someone commit suicide by hanging, and this as well as her father's demise had affected her disposition. Since she was usually quite cheerful, there was the possibility that the discarnate entity from the hanging suicide might have attached to her, and imprinted on her. She had tried to hang herself several times. Later it transpired there had been two unnatural deaths in the family, which may have influenced her.

When the psychiatrist asked an occultist to look at her energetically he confirmed she had an imprint: they were asked to remove the pattern from her. Dr Basu explained: *"she saw a suicide in childhood, and later had depressive spells. These childhood memories leave their impressions and I believe that such cases might also benefit from occult help in addition to western psychiatric treatment. We are developing trials in some cases like this, where together with our psychiatric interventions, occult practices from experts have been recommended (like praying, burning camphor, and use of special stones charged with power etc)."*

From the above cases, it seemed Dr Basu's treatment for his female patient with the young baby, was to offer the appropriate psychiatric pharmacology, suggest a religious ritual to clear the air in the house, say prayers at a local shrine, and pragmatically, to dispose of artefacts that had a negative history attached. In the second case a healer also offered advice. There were other cases where he worked with traditional healers who referred patients on to him. *"I found that people who are practicing shamanism, who are practicing occult healing, they also felt that some of the patients should be seen by doctors. In our special geographical place where I work, this type of occult healer, Muslims and Hindus, they somehow prefer me, and they started sending me patients, telling them that 'we have done our occult work, now this has to be supplemented by some medicines, and you go to this doctor, he will give you the required medicines".*

Dr Basu came to regard healers in a non-judgmental way. They wanted to help, would observe patients sitting in the clinic, and say *'they all need your help, but one needs extra help from us'."* He joined our conversation but changed the topic and presented us with a different insight on murder and spirit possession: *"if a man committed murder, there was no point in punishing him or carrying out the death penalty, without addressing the spirit that possessed him, and forced him to carry out the murder. If the possessing spirit was not healed, it would jump onto someone else, and force them to commit future dark deeds".* He explained we needed to lift the occupying spirit to allow real healing change to occur, and stop the pattern of murder. Compassion and prayer were said to be the way forward.

Dr Pandey added that he felt there was a problem when medical practitioners had reduced awareness of other beings in existence, and he considered this could result in prolonging someone's mental distress: *"Our ignorance also hinders true intervention. We really don't know what is happening. We stem peoples' consciousness with drugs, but the being or the fragment of the being remains, or their consciousness remains at the same level, so there is a tendency for illnesses to reoccur, or to be prolonged."*

SUMMARY

What did all these beliefs mean for health care?
The concept of an individual self, which could be
overshadowed by a disembodied being, meant
when mental illness occurred in India, it was less an
individual's responsibility. Also, if there were specialists
in occult vision, it seemed patients also considered
consulting them. In the ashram some practitioners
thought that perhaps due to the 'unseen' beings, humans
should have mastery over physical, mental and emotional
health, in order not to attract them. Mental stability I
was told, was clearly important, because without it, one
could not do Sri Aurobindo's yoga, nor receive any kind
of spiritual force. I wondered whether there were people
who felt the 'spiritual force' but couldn't contain it. This
may be like the so-called spiritual emergencies described
by psychiatrist Stan Grof in California[62].

In this chapter I covered esoteric explanatory models for
mental distress. The material was based on interviews
with psychiatrists, homoeopaths, a medical herbalist and
lay people. Interviewees mentioned the role of planetary
influences, past lives, and subtle energies like the 'force'
which was said to be around the samadhi in Pondicherry.

Spirit possession was explored and I was told ways in which disembodied beings might be created. A cautionary note was expressed by one interviewee about the dangers of intense practices as a possible trigger for mental illness. Several individuals suggested a relationship between spiritual practice and psychotic experience.

PART FOUR

INDIAN FRAMEWORKS OF KNOWLEDGE

Chapter Ten

PHILOSOPHIES
OF PSYCHOLOGY

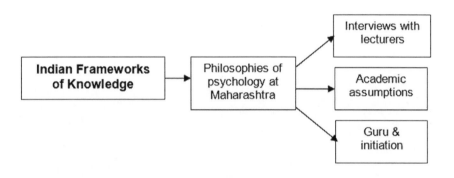

Introduction

Within western cultural psychiatry there has been an underlying assumption people with functional mental health problems are influenced by post-natal experiences. However, this is less frequently the case in India, where I met psychiatrists and psychologists, educated according to western medical models, who took account of many different influences on their patients' health including pre-natal.

In this chapter, in order to investigate eastern and western frameworks of knowledge in more depth, I travelled to Maharashtra to interview two Indian lecturers of psychology, and talked with them of their concerns about cultural awareness. I wanted to hear about their cultural frameworks for understanding mental distress and addressing human suffering.

Discussions based on interviews with staff, brought out their fears about the under-acknowledgement of Indian philosophy and psychology in academia, as well as lecturers' frustrations at having to meet western exam board requirements of teaching philosophy, which did not incorporate their students' life experiences.

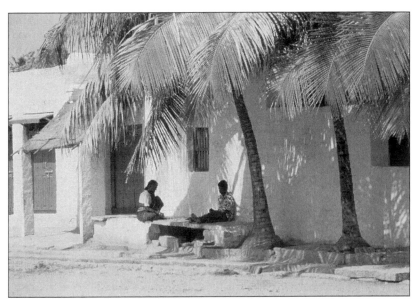

Journey through Karnataka, photo by Jean-Pierre Ribière

Journey to Solapur, Maharashtra

I travelled by train to Solapur to meet Dr Mistry, a surgeon and homoeopathic, who was a devotee of Sri Aurobindo, but lived in his home village. On the train, I had a seat in a deluxe first class carriage. I shared this most expensive train compartment with two men: it cost a stunning 3,000 rupees for the overnight journey. There was red carpet on the floor, a covered sink and tap by the window, and a plastic waste-bin emptied by staff several times during the journey. The fittings and seats were of red and black embroidery. There were textile curtains over the windows and doors, with foliate designs on them. This air conditioned cabin was extra wide, with a mirror, bottle holders and shelves. All the bedding was provided: two white sheets, a clean cotton pillow, a woollen blanket, and a towel.

As we travelled from Chennai through Andra Pradesh and Karnataka I reminded myself that several years earlier I had conducted research there, as a guest of Achyutadevaraya, descendant of the Kings of Vijayanagara. I had then written a book on indigenous architecture in a royal village[63]. I was familiar with these states and yet I felt I was travelling through them as if for the first time, as if I had never been there before.

Dr Mistry was waiting for me on the platform when the train arrived at Solapur station. In the town, traffic seemed less frenetic than Pondicherry or Kolkata, with slower and more considerate driving: there was a less thrusting energy. People were simply travelling, not rushing to get anywhere. I felt as if I was somewhere different: the architecture was more Islamic, the town hall completely Islamic in style. There were lots of Muslim women in full veil, or with just their eyes showing. There were few westerners here. We stopped in the market: there was plenty of fresh produce, sweet fruits, and vibrant coloured vegetables.

On the gates of his house was an old rusty sign saying "Dr Mistry surgeon and homoeopath". Inside was a garden full of plants, trees and shrubs. Dr Mistry was chief editor of the Homoeopathic Clinical Case Recorder[64] published in Maharashtra. He had invited me to stay with him and his wife, and he introduced me to teachers of philosophy and to one of his own gurus, so that I would learn more about philosophies of psychology and personal realisation.

His homoeopathic clinic started at 9.00 am, and before then people sat and waited outside in the garden. Seated on stone benches and woven beds, trained assistants took the patients' case histories. Dr Mistry asked his patients to stay with him for life and not swing back and forwards between homoeopathy and allopathy. He did however suggest they use allopathic diagnostic tests for blood and urine to support the diagnostic process. A patient's case history of life events and body malfunctions were taken into account and recorded by assistants: I was told unsettled emotions could result in biological cell damage.

Lecturer of Philosophy

The day after my arrival Dr Mistry introduced me to Professor Katkar, a gentleman teacher approaching retirement, with a Masters in Philosophy[65]. Since 1974 he had been a lecturer in philosophy in Solapur in the same college as Dr Mistry's wife. I looked forward to meeting this scholar, whose forefathers had been court advisors in Karnataka to Raja Krishnadevaraya of Vijayanagara in the 15th century. We walked to his house with its narrow ground floor base, built upwards on several floors. We sat in the yellow painted veranda, all harmonious shades of yellow, ochre and brown. Even his shirt was pale yellow. He gave sermons in a hall in the upper storey of his home. He held public gatherings and discussions every day except Monday on 'systems of knowledge and human experience'.

Professor Katkar questioned whether our original knowledge base could be expanded to what was beyond the five senses, which had been so empirically explored by science. He felt there was a gap between what his students were tested on, for the academic disciplines of philosophy and psychology, and their actual experiences within Indian culture. We were joined later during the discussion by a couple of his colleagues including Dr Suneet, a lecturer in philosophy at Delhi University, who was interested in the evolution of consciousness[66].

The psychiatrist Dr Basu had already made me aware within western psychiatry there was an underlying assumption people with mental health problems were only influenced by post-natal experiences. Although there were exceptions in UK[67]: professionals who considered transpersonal aspects of their patients' experiences, or places which offered university degrees. However, in India, more professionals, practitioners and lay people were familiar with other models of psychology, which took account of pre-natal experiences and survival beyond death.

Sitting comfortably in the cool veranda, I asked Professor Katkar whether there was a correlation between the kind of philosophy he taught at the college, and lay people's knowledge, and their human experience of life. "*The teaching of philosophy we do at university is totally unrelated to our spiritual life in India. It is totally irrelevant. There is not simply a gap in the knowledge there is a sort of opposition. We are habituated to think that there is something beyond our physical senses. So nowadays what we teach as philosophy, it has no relation with our spiritual experiences or our aspiration.*"

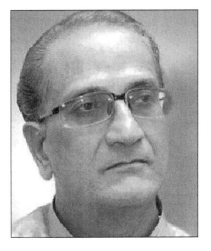

Professor Katkar

I was surprised at the vehemence of his comment, from such a mild mannered gentleman. He continued *"What am I to do with my spiritual experiences if I am taught a philosophy of Derrida, post modernism, or Descartes. What Kirkegaard says about fear, falling aside from divinity, negation of the self: we Hindus can understand what he says about fear, miseries of life, despair, but how is it possible for us to know about things from a spiritual view about Wittgenstein, about Russell, who says human knowledge is limited to the empirical sphere. We teach them Kant, Jung, Hegel, Greek philosophy, and mediaeval European philosophy."*

I asked whether he felt the philosophy curriculum he taught was culture bound. Did he feel it was based on a western system of understanding, and a western knowledge base? *"At present what we teach as philosophy is predominantly a western philosophy. In my undergraduate class, my teaching begins with Greek philosophy and not the Indian philosophy. Now what relevance is this to Indian students of 17 or 18 years of age? Of course there are perennial questions, I agree, which transcend culture and nationality and race. But still we must take into consideration the differences of life experiences."*

He considered the education system needed to take a hard look at itself, to explore its own underlying assumptions, to see what it called knowledge, and to see the topics it tested and examined as knowledge. He thought there was a similar issue within psychiatry and psychology. *"In psychology, the same question arises. The treatment given by an American psychiatrist to his patient will be totally different from the treatment given by an Indian psychiatrist to his Indian patient.*

A system that is termed abnormal in America need not be abnormal here in our culture."

"These differences exist, within psychiatry, psychology or philosophy. For example hearing music, where no one is playing, may be treated as a symptom of schizophrenia by western psychiatry, but an Indian doctor may think that there is some ghost or spirit in contact with the person. Perhaps we may say that the Indian doctor is unscientific, but his own scientific treatment is Indian, for he may prescribe a lower dose, and it may work. If it works and a person becomes free of their symptoms, this means we need change to a result-oriented outlook."

Professor Katkar explained until recently scientific analysis had only been based on the five senses. Those people like the shaman or clairvoyant, who saw beyond the five senses, considered what they saw to be a truth, but for someone who couldn't see, it was an untruth. It depended on the observer's perception and sensitivity. For someone who could see beyond, then a visionary event may be veridical, the truth, but for someone who was unable to see, it appeared to be a fantasy or a delusion. He considered there was a lack of understanding in the west, that human beings had different faculties and abilities. There was more than one possible framework for understanding events. There were different ways of seeing.

Professor Katkar continued: *"an Indian would look at shamanism as a natural thing. This belief is ingrained in us, that there is something beyond that which we experience with our five senses. It is an intrinsic belief for an Indian, that there is something beyond. So if someone claims that there is something beyond which is influencing their life, the Indian will take it as something very natural."*

He was sad that academia had set its own boundaries for knowledge. *"Whether it is western academia or Indian, academics have made some presuppositions; that what we see is the only reality, what we experience through our sense organs is the only reality, that there is nothing beyond. This is a presupposition which they have taken for granted, and are not prepared, mentally or intellectually to set it aside."*

Listening to his arguments, I invited him to consider what he would do, if he was given the opportunity to redesign the curriculum for philosophy. *"I am sure that I will not be allowed to change the curriculum, but if the chance is given to me I will go directly to the common man. I will ask about his expectations, how he views his life, who he is, and what he thinks about the world, about his family members, and what he thinks about the reality of the relation you have taken for granted. From his ordinary language, I will develop the philosophy. Each philosophy if it is to be genuine must have grounding in the aspirations of common individuals. Let us not compartmentalise what is material, and what is spiritual."*

"We say 'purushastra', that means 'ideas of human beings'. It is not that we want worldly pleasures. We want prosperity, but at the same time we want to remain in this life, and go beyond life, in accordance with some divine law. That aspiration to live in accordance with divine law is called dharma. At the same time, we want to free ourselves from all the miseries of this life, and that is called moksha."

Based on what he was saying there appeared to be a fundamental difference of understanding, where students of one culture were being examined according to the knowledge base of another culture, and the two frameworks of knowledge were not connected. He explained that the student's understanding, which was developed from being examined on western cultural grounds was totally false. I wondered whether the same situation was developing in Europe, when we taught and examined students according to a materialist knowledge base of reality, when their actual human experience went beyond that. Would an existential confusion develop within them?

Professor Katkar thought problems would develop, and gave an example: "*Skinner was an American psychologist, who totally integrated the concept of consciousness. Suppose there is a psychologist who belongs to the behaviourist school, he will just treat his patient for having behavioural maladjustment. He won't think there is a soul, or some disturbance in the soul itself. He will give some tablets, but the problem won't be solved.* Dr Mistry joined in the conversation and explained what he felt would happen in these circumstances: "*the patient who is treated will get such a wrong treatment, and he will get worse, or end up in a mental hospital. The treatment will do the opposite, and it may cause a total break down at all levels.*"

What it was like I wondered, for Professor Katkar to teach philosophy in a university, and offer a subject whose course content he felt was inappropriate to the lives of his students? How could he do this when at the same time he knew there was a culturally appropriate philosophy of existence within grasp, but not examinable within the curriculum timetable? He replied concisely: "*My situation is this; when I teach, I feel I'm teaching something very superficial. It has no connexion with the student's soul nor with their individuality. I teach because I need the salary.*"

"*In ancient times philosophy was taught in India, in ashrams. We were taught that we were not this body, we were brahman, and so we didn't fear death... You see the philosophy and the human situation are correlated. There is a person who is afraid of death and there is the teacher. The master teaches him not to be afraid of death, for it belongs to the body, but we are beyond the body. The teaching correlates with the needs of the person. Today there is no correlation between teaching and pupils. There are different models, motivated by different ideals, and the philosophy we teach them has no correlation with their ideals.*"

Academic Assumptions and Hierarchies of Knowledge

At that point in our discussions, Professor Katkar's wife ushered in a tall younger man: this was Dr Suneet who for a short time joined us in our discussion on the veranda. He was a lecturer in a university in Delhi in the philosophy of psychology, and interested in consciousness studies. After greetings were exchanged and we sat drinking cool pomegranate juice, I wanted to know whether he felt the same way, and asked him how he managed to integrate Indian psychology within the philosophy courses he taught.

He told me: *"We have promoted a psychology, which doesn't have much to offer our society, so I am trying to promote a psychology, which is appropriate to India. I delineate the hegemony of western ideas, using the category of science and projecting it as the knowledge. I deconstruct that, and show the links between power and knowledge. I pave the way for discourses on reality. I expand on India's systems of psychology (including Vedanta and Buddhist). This allows me to touch on all the key issues in the debate. I call it 'the quest for appropriate psychology'"*.

On the topic of mental health, I wondered whether Dr Suneet could outline any differences he had found between western and Indian psychology. He explained there were several major themes that were different from the western tradition. *"The western approach, being the medical model, is based on classification of diseases, with strict categories as found in the DSM. Mostly within the academic world, our students are taught the western model. Somewhere as a footnote, it is mentioned that there are certain Indian approaches. But these approaches are not taken up in detail nor in any systematic manner in our university departments"*.

"Some individuals like myself are interested in these non-western approaches. I have come across several approaches, which are not in the academic university system. They are mostly outside it. Although that is not to say that they are not happening in the west, such as Buddhist psychotherapy. These insights and approaches are a big phenomena in the west, in Europe, and United States. However in India they are not taught as psychology."

"Another approach is looking at mental illness as spirit possession. In north India where I come from, this is practiced in the villages. There, a priest or shaman would be called to a house where individuals are possessed, and put the spirit to rest. This is one of several practices. There is one Balaji temple in north India, in Rajesthan. That is the place where Sudhir Kakar[68] carried out his study, but his interpretation was largely psycho-analytic. He looked at the phenomena through the eyes of a psychoanalyst, and then fitted things into that system."

"But in the villages and in these temples, they are not aware of psychoanalysis and they don't practise it. But what they do, works, and people benefit. Most of the people benefit and the person suffering becomes all right. 'All right' in quotes, since we have to start by saying what we mean by 'all right'. One attributes that to a different cause altogether, some kind of negative force or some kind of evil spirit. This is one tradition not taught in the universities."

He told us when he was studying for his PhD, he experienced resistance within his department when he said he wanted to do it on the topic of "eastern psychology". I asked him how as a lecturer he presented the topic within the curriculum. *"I explore mainstream academic psychology as the psychology of a particular cultural group. Then I address the psychologies which are derived within an Indian context. I emphasise that Buddhism is explicitly a system of dealing with human suffering, and I believe suffering is largely psychological suffering. Buddhism starts with the premise that there is suffering in the world. There is a reason for it, a way out of it, and it tells us the way out. If this is not psychotherapy, then I don't know what is. It is most explicitly psychology and dealing with mental health, and how to attain mental health[69]."*

"However, in India it is not part of the academic system, to study centres where people go to be helped. It is a system in practice in India, but not in the academic world. It is not recognised by the academicians. The following are western categories: philosophy and religion, psychology, ways of living. In India these categories collapse: they all fuse into one. In earlier times, psychology only meant a particular kind of psychology. But the Post Modern turn in Social Sciences, which allows for cultural constructions of reality, included cultural constructions of psychic reality, mind as constituted by society or culture."

He explained to us his opinion on the unequal hierarchies of knowledge, and how he responded to it as an academic. *"The politics of knowledge disturb me and I do not wish to be part of the system where we are victims, so I choose to publish here. I refused to publish in western journals. The main reason is that we have developed a blind faith in the efficacy of science and psychoanalytic psychology. We have developed a sense of inferiority. We believe that western society is superior, in its ability to think and act rationally, and modern science is a reflection of that, and it is the only way to progress. We have the terms: developed world and developing world. In India many of us have found that this path does not necessarily lead to a better world, even in the west."*

Understanding Western Perspectives in India

I was told about some research that took place in India and was reported in 2006[70]. The aim was to test the effect of education about biomedical interventions for psychosis against the indigenous beliefs and explanatory models of 80 female community health workers in Vellore, Tamil Nadu.

After two weeks training, the indigenous beliefs were tested again. One of the conclusions was that educational intervention can change the explanatory models of mental illness among health workers, and they were more likely to describe symptoms of psychosis using bio-medical explanations. Although the researchers recognised local cultural perceptions were important, it looked as if their underlying assumption was biomedical approaches were more appropriate for early recognition and treatment of symptoms.

That research was followed by another study[71], also in Vellore, which acknowledged that multiple contradictory bio-medical and indigenous beliefs were held simultaneously, and people sought help from each health system at the same time. I am wondering if there is a problem, when healthcare practitioners who hold multiple explanatory models, are taught there is only one model for understanding health. What kinds of dissonance might there be between their culture of origin, and their clinical training?

In America, Yale University conducted an empirical investigation of mental health clinicians' ontological beliefs about mental disorders. It discovered that clinicians treated conditions differently: ontological beliefs had implications for clinicians' beliefs about the effectiveness of psychotherapy or medication, and therefore their choice of treatment options[72]. These studies indicating the moving relationship between knowledge and belief, are surely an argument for wide ranging training in cultural awareness and self reflection?

Divine Masters

Our discussions gave me much to think about. Both men taught philosophy, and each was aware from an academic perspective, Indian psychology had little role to play in the curriculum. However the younger lecturer had found ways of incorporating it, so his students could discuss the varieties of different systems. Superficially it seemed as though colonial attitudes towards knowledge still influenced the content of material taught in Indian universities. However, I wondered whether this was really a case of colonial paradigm blindness, or if it went deeper, and was about core beliefs about the nature of human existence.

As discussions drew to a close, we accepted some tea and sweet biscuits, which Mrs Katkar prepared for us and continued our discussion with talk about possession states, temple healing, and occult practitioners. Shortly afterwards Dr Suneet left the house to attend another meeting, but Dr Mistry and I continued to talk with Professor Katkar until dusk fell.

I asked Professor Katkar to help me understand why people in India took gurus and masters, and received initiation. I wanted to further explore their role in initiation and in spiritual well-being and health. Due to his daily sermons and university teaching Professor Katkar was familiar with aspects of life concerning masters, initiation and personal health and he started to answer my questions from his perspective. *"Masters are in a sense, representatives of the divine upon this earth. They are both divine in themselves, and representatives of the divine. The divine is something beyond my human nature, so there must be some sort of connecting link between myself and divinity. This could be a guru or master as a connecting link. They will bring down the divine force, back to us. They will lift us, from our thoughts, our impunity."*

"The role of initiation, of genuine initiation must work in a twofold way. It should bring down the divine force to the person being initiated. At the same time all their human limitations should spontaneously or gradually vanish, and they become as similar as possible to the divine being. That is the role of initiation, a genuine initiation (diksha). The contact between master and pupil (shisha) is everlasting."

I had heard the term 'realised being' in connection with Sri Ramana Maharshi, the guru at Tiruvanamalai, but I wasn't really sure what it meant. Professor Katkar explained: *"the term 'realisation' can be defined in so many ways, but it is a state, which can be obtained at different levels; physical, mental, and intellectual. These levels pertain to different aspects of our personality. You must become free from limitations, at the level at which the realisation takes place. For example at the physical level, limitations must spontaneously vanish or go gradually."*

"This will affect your health and ill health, but the extent that it works depends on so many factors, depending on the person who has the initiation, their karma, and their future spiritual progress. There are so many factors, which decide the extent to which a person may be cured from physical and mental illness."

I wondered whether it was the same for mental and emotional health, and intellectual stability. *"Gradually wholesome results should permeate. The divine force should permeate the whole individual, and gradually individuality must transform. Realisation at the cellular level means a sort of healing or resistance to the forces that create ill health. The whole personality will be divinised."*

I asked if he would tell me about spiritual well-being. *"Spiritual well-being is a continuous communion with the divine. You must feel divine by being divine. This is what I have understood by spiritual realisation: both communion and identification with the divine. Divine presence is with me. It is not only beyond, it is also here. It is within me, and it is also beyond me."* I was told initiation with a master would bring about a level of divine realisation that would dissolve mental distress and alleviate physical illness. I wanted to understand more about initiation.

Ground Roots Guru and Initiation

Dr Mistry and I thanked our host Professor Katkar for his detailed explanations and his hospitality. We walked back to his house, planning our visit to a guru the following day. Dr Mistry had offered to take me after the clinic, to meet one of his gurus in a nearby ashram just outside Solapur. This was to help me learn about initiation and the existence of those who renounce mundane life.

We travelled by car to the ashram to meet the guru, with Dr Mistry at the wheel. The drive to the *Math* (ashram) was through the sandy dry lands of Maharashtra, on a small track, off the main road. After one and a half hours we reached a small a village with very simple houses. Next door was the Math, a highly painted building, constructed on various levels.

In one room we found Swamiji sitting on a tiger skin edged with orange cloth. In his late 60's, he was entirely dressed in orange robes. A renunciate, he had a long white beard, long hair, a plump face and persistently smiling eyes. He smiled the whole time, smiling from the depth of his being.

Dr Mistry explained the significance of the colour orange for sanyasin: *"This is a uniform of renunciation and is a symbol of the renunciate. This is the dress of Lord Vishnu Narayan. This colour means everything is surrendered to the Lord. You have nothing of your own. When they take these robes, of a sanyasin, everything in their previous life is supposed to be burnt. After the ceremonies, there is no other life but total surrender to the lord."*

"Swamiji had already done his death ceremonies when he got his sanyasin initiation. I cannot wear this colour, I would have to take the sanyas for this, and I don't want to. It is nice to be a family man: it is nice to be small. Never become a guru! Even he would not like to be a guru!! The lord gave him permission otherwise he would still be just a devotee. For 40 years he was a sadhak, then the lord gave consent and he became a guru. Unless the lord said, he couldn't do it. If you become a guru on your own, then alas, so many people have slipped! They deceive us and they deceive themselves. The Lord or Divine Mother has to give consent."

"This place is called Sri Guru dev Sidha Ashram, at the village of Degaon. It is an ashram for all realised gurus. Lord Rama has been at this place and the rishis and sages of that particular time had been here since then, thousands of years ago. This place was an ashram for the rishis for thousands of years, and they are still here. Lord Rama's footsteps are here. These people are not healers: they are holders of the divine force."

He told me Swamiji had been at this Math for 55 years. I asked whether he always knew he would have a life here from this birth and now at this Math, or did he have some other life before? Did he have some other kind of work before this, in this lifetime? *"He has come definitely for this purpose only. The work he had to do, and the kind of knowledge he needed was given to him at the age of nine. A spiritual master known as aulia (that is a God realised person) proclaimed his mission when he was five years old and then in his ninth year it started. He is from here, born here in this village. His family is here. He was born Hindu of a Marathi family, but now there is no Hindu,*

Muslim, or Christian religion. Once he takes sanyas, all religious things are pushed aside. This is not a question of religion, it is divine force."

Meditation room. Swamiji greeted us, and showed us around different rooms in the Math. One was constructed over a cave where the original *rishi* used to meditate. *"Swamiji is the present incarnation of Lord Paddaturi, the guru of gurus who has taken birth. This is his meditation room. That is where he sits. He is inviting you to sit down."* I sat in the place where he usually sat and closed my eyes. He put his hand on my forehead between my eyes and tapped my head. Suddenly I saw an ephemeral white being come up from the chamber below into the room where we were sitting, with his form being in both chambers, his head above in the room with us. *"That rishi is from Lord Rama's side: he can give you his presence, either through touch or through a light form."*

Swamiji continued to press my forehead. *"Close your eyes for one minute, and I'll close mine."* I saw an ephemeral deep blue being, in the same room as us, in the corner. *"That was the female energy, Shakti. Swamiji had a ritual performed on him by Tibetan masters, and as a result of that, as a gift, that particular feminine energy was given, to be with him permanently. What you saw there, the blue being, was the feminine energy, and the white form was the rishi's energy, masculine energy. The rishi is a sage or a realised being."* The beings I had been allowed to see, I was told had both come from Tibet.

I was surprised: it was decades since I had allowed any 'seeing'. I thought that side of me had closed down, as I had forbidden it. I asked Dr Mistry whether the energies of the deities and ephemeral light beings came through Swamiji, and then appeared to the people attending. *"Yes that is right, when he was in Tibet certain things were given to him as a special gift from the Tibetan masters. Then when he came back here, he percolated their particular energy and spread it. Now on every no-moon day, when he does a particular ritual or puja, he takes a certain amount of energy and gives it to the fire. Through the medium of Agni (fire, the first God of the cosmos) all the other energies are brought into him, and then focussed onto or into the person concerned."*

We moved through another chamber, up some steps to a veranda where we sat drinking sweet tea, shaded by a cloth canopy. Swamiji, still smiling, sitting cross-legged on a rug said I could ask him any questions. Dr Mistry translated. I asked whether he would help me understand the concepts of initiation and realisation. *"There are three stages: in Sanskrit, diksha, amukra, sat-sat-kar. When there is initiation (diksha), the master concerned makes your energies inside active, so you are aware of them. Those energies, normally present inside each of us, are awakened through the process of initiation. Then there is a higher process: what swamiji has got inside him, he can awaken in you. This energy he can put into another person's body. That is a higher form of initiation. First is diksha, then is amukra, after that is realisation (sat-sat-kar). You will get that as a pupil."*

"Then you become one with the universe, with energy, light, or cosmos. When you get realisation in a body, you get a universal feeling, but you still remain. That is when you get realisation in the body. Once you drop the body, there are two choices; to completely go inside universal, your individuality will be gone. If you want to come back for a purpose after that particular stage, you take a rest for some time, then you use will-power and thought to come back with full knowledge."

We were shown around another chamber, which contained two samadhi (tomb or resting places) from the seven original residents of this place. In one, the occupant took a living death with permission of the king, and was covered over whilst still alive and conscious. The other occupants had died before being placed. Dr Mistry explained: *"These are the samadhis of swamiji's spiritual predecessors. This man took a living samadhi. He didn't die. He went inside and he did certain rituals (kriyas), and they covered up the samadhi, and his consciousness stayed. That is living samadhi. It is not because you have passed away they put the body there. It was his choice. If you can see with the inner eye, you will still find him sitting inside. He had special permission to take a living samadhi. All the great masters know their time of departure, to the second and minute. Before they pass away, they have already prepared their place. As soon as they pass away, their body is immediately put in the designated space."*

"After him, Swamiji is the 8ᵗʰ in this line, the last resident. His potential spot is already prepared, in advance. When he goes, they will put him inside and the whole thing will be covered up. The ground has already been prepared for his mortal remains. His own samadhi has already been built. He knows exactly where he will be located in death. There will be no others after him."

"You see that carved stone tortoise set in the ground? The meaning of the tortoise is that it has the capacity to take all his limbs inside, and when he wants, he can bring them out. This is Swamiji's natural abilities. He has got the capacity to take his senses inside and to remove the outer senses. That is why it is the symbol of the last one."

"When Swamiji's incarnate life is over, and he takes samadhi, does part of his awareness stay here?" *"The energies, those which he brought for this world, all those energies will remain here in that samadhi. But he will be liberated, in a different dimension, and he will not be connected with his body."*

Before we left, Swamiji showed us around a chamber containing an everlasting fire-pit: in the morning the fire subsided, and in the night it grew. The ceremonies around this fire at the ashram had been conducted for 700 years. *"The fire is always in a stable state. It has never gone out. Not one day has it ever gone out. And every no moon day, Swamiji performs a particular ritual. People come and book to be here months in advance. After the ceremonies for two or three years, all the energies of all the gods are invoked by him, to bless people who have come."*

As we left Swamiji gave me some ash from the sacred fire pit, for my mother who had been feeling unwell.

He suggested that for seven days she should eat a pinch of it in the evenings, and apply some of it to her body and then she would notice the difference with her health. I don't know if she tried it, but although my mother has since died, I have retained to this day a small amount of that ash.

SUMMARY

I had had marvellous experiences and met lecturers of philosophy and psychology who expressed frustration at the academic system, and the failure of their exam system set in UK, that didn't appear to respect local practices. I'd learnt about transpersonal psychological approaches which were common practice in the west but were not taught as part of the Indian curriculum. Hierarchies of knowledge that were based in western philosophy did not appear to acknowledge Indian practices of psychology in India. I had wondered whether academic restrictions were part of colonial blindness or part of a deeper western denial about existential realities.

Our discussions with Dr Mistry and Swamiji about masters and gurus had given me insight into concepts of realisation and divinity, and I learnt some masters were not healers but rather they were holders of divine force. They had a different role in life, and in death.

Dr Mistry and I drove back to Solapur and I said goodbye to his family. I left Maharashtra and their hospitable kindness, and travelled onwards by train: another overnight journey. As the train rattled along the tracks towards Tamil Nadu in South India, I wondered how the life experiences of one guru in the small village of Degaon compared to the experiences of the sage Sri Aurobindo and the thousands of devotes at his ashram in Pondicherry.

In Pondicherry I intended to talk to medical and health care professionals about their philosophies and knowledge frameworks for interpreting health and well being. I stayed for some weeks, talking to practitioners about different healing therapies and modalities, and their understanding of layers of consciousness described by the sage Sri Aurobindo

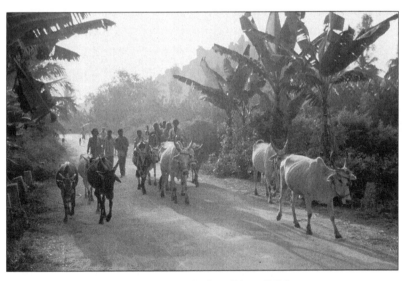

Drylands, photo by Jean-Pierre Ribière

Chapter Eleven

PHILOSOPHIES OF HEALTH

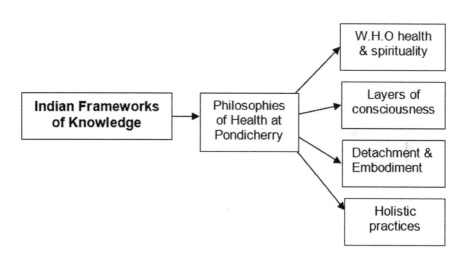

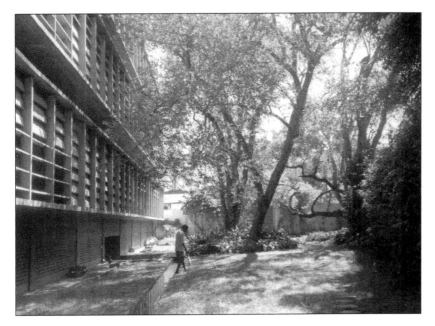

Residences at Golconde

Lodgings in Pondicherry

I got off the train and took a taxi from the station to the ashram residence known as Golconde. The clairvoyant photographer Viswajt had introduced me to people who ran this ashramite residence for visitors, and a place was offered to me in that peaceful haven. An English woman in her 90's whose family came from Essex had been in charge. She was feisty, and vetted anyone who went there. When a devotee arrived, they were given a small booklet entitled: "Golconde", which was printed by the Sri Aurobindo Ashram Press. Inside was written "*being a resident at Golconde is a privilege, a responsibility, and an opportunity*".

The booklet said; "*it is not a guest house, it is a house on which Mother placed 'Her Consciousness Force'*. People who stayed there were selected. They were '*the right people*', '*trained to a less rough and ready living than is common*'. Those who stayed must be '*worthy of the privilege*'. There were a set of 29 recommendations in the booklet, about how the room should be kept, how to use the shutters, about the use of food and water in the room, laundry, visitors, and the presence of servants, typewriters and radios.

I was shown a room on the first floor, with wood panelling inner walls and concrete slats to allow air through. It faced onto the garden and in the afternoons I could see shimmering reflections of sunlight on the ceiling from the surrounding channels of water. The windows and outer walls of the entire building were of slatted concrete, which could be angled or closed. I left my umbrella and my street shoes downstairs in a numbered rack. My laundry had to be put out by 6am each morning, neatly wrapped with the wooden room number badge on top. Washing of laundry was not allowed in the rooms or in wash-basins. The toilets and bathrooms were communal, shared by whoever was resident on that floor. I signed in and out every time I arrived or left. There were no locks on the door, just on the wardrobe inside. At 3.00pm each day a cup of tea was offered to residents in the garden.

During torrential monsoon rains, it was an austere building, with the concrete shutters closed. The inner walls were made of woven strips of wood, polished brown with wax. The toilets, showers and washbasins were spotlessly clean. It was a privilege to be offered a place there. All my clothes were washed and ironed. The furniture in the room had to be maintained in the correct position. If I moved the footstool, and placed it beside my bed, once the room was cleaned it was returned to its place by the chair. My pen was placed straight on the desk. In the evening I had a hot shower. It was such a luxury for me: I was used to washing from a bucket of water, sometimes warm, sometimes not.

My room was beside the garden, and I kept the shutters open. The garden was exquisite: it had such a sense of peace and serenity. There were tiny birds among the sparse foliage of the tree. On the rockery were snakes and darting dragonflies. A kingfisher sat on a branch, then flew with its long red beak, turquoise wings, and black and white under-body. It swooped from the branch into the water channel below, in order to catch one of the thousands of tiny fish swimming there. In the evenings I sat and transcribed my interview notes by the light of a single lamp, burning incense sticks to protect myself from mosquitoes.

In the night, when it rained again I heard a chorus of frogs, together with the wind blowing through the trees. When I got up, there was a thin ghostly figure at the end of the corridor, walking silently to the bathroom. I had met this elderly Indian lady on other evenings, shivering in the corridor in her diaphanous sari and shawl, in this place that was so draughty in the cold weather. She walked quietly like a ghostly shadow in the dark corridor.

The Beach Office

During the day, I helped out occasionally at the Beach Office, editing articles for their journal NAMAH (New Approaches to Medicine and Health). The medical team in the Beach Office were in a department of Sri Aurobindo's Ashram, known as the Academy of the Future. The modern white painted offices were the headquarters of SAIIIHR (Sri Aurobindo International Institute for Integrated Health Research). These offices with a large conference hall were built along the seashore, overlooking the promenade.

Over the years things changed: the co-ordinator's chambers were at the outskirts of town, whereas the homoeopathic team had moved independently to cool, bright modern chambers on the beach road, facing the sea.

Spirituality

The World Health Organisation

The Sri Aurobindo International Institute for Integral Health and Research (SAIIIHR) was established in 1992, with Dr Bisht as Chair. Their aim was to explore paradigms of health and psychology from a consciousness perspective. This group felt although modern medicine had developed unparalleled achievements in the field of specialist research, there were various human issues that could not be explained from a mechanistic perspective. They believed a deeper understanding of the manifestations of ill-health could be found in the philosophies of Sri Aurobindo, who considered consciousness predated the manifestation of matter, and was the essence inherent in all reality.

Staff at SAHIIIR considered spirituality was crucial, and people were 'persons not patients'. During a first appointment, a person's history was taken, and considered essential before clinicians prescribed. With regard to spiritual beliefs about holism and the totality of human existence, the underlying assumption was that when one died in this life that was not the end. Staff explained *"No Indian person will believe that their physical problem is only physical. They might want a physical cure for it. But if the problem persists, everyone knows there could be a karmic background to it, and so the problem has to be worked out either by a priest or someone who is spiritual. In India we don't have divisions between spirit, religion, and the physical body.*" Many of the doctors at the centre agreed with this and felt there was a role for non-physical or spiritual factors affecting health, which went beyond mind and emotions.

One day I had a chat with Dr Bisht who had worked with the World Health Organisation and was then Chair of the Sri Aurobindo International Institute. He had learnt about the philosophy of Sri Aurobindo after he'd got a job in Pondicherry, and had served as the Mother's physician. He was interested in spirituality and health: *"In 1978, when I was the Director General of health, I represented India on WHO's executive board. I thought their definition of health was incomplete if we did not add the spiritual dimension to it. I felt there should be some difference between the definition of animal health and human health. Human health had to have something more. Something more had to be added to WHO's own definition of health. This was accepted by a resolution in WHO in 1982, and in 1983, it became obligatory to include spiritual health in WHO's directives".*

"That health is a positive sense of well-being, physical, mental, social, and spiritual (and not merely the absence of disease or infirmity): that 'spiritual' word was added because of my efforts. In 1998 WHO took up my recommendation, and it was validated. After I retired from Director General of health of India, I joined WHO as deputy regional director for the whole of South East Asia. I retired in 1994. After I retired, I came here, and three days later I wrote up the entire SAHIIIR thing with Vijay. The society passed a resolution and agreed to it."

I asked Dr Bisht his opinions about concepts of health based on the assumption that a person only lives once, and when the physical body dies, the whole person dies. These are the beliefs of some people in the health systems of the western world. Did he think there was any problem with medical training based on that premise or perception? "*There are different ways of looking at it. We are continually moving from the material world to the philosophical to the world beyond matter. The physical world is dominated by physical forces; we are affected by gravity, light, and electricity. They can alter the physical status of the body. We know that there are mental forces. A psychiatrist knows spiritual forces can make some changes here. Similarly socio-economic forces can affect health.*"

"*Lack of health does not mean ill health. It is a very thin line. So health and ill health must be understood in their correct perspectives. Biological health is only the physical and vital combined. Humanity in the course of time is progressing, and probably it will reach the highest level of the Supramental consciousness possible, ultimately reaching God or the divine or whatever. The causes of mental ill health are the actions of the forces of mental health. One can manifest one's own thoughts to cause mental ill health, or outer forces can affect it.*"

Dr Bisht said he had talked about a spiritual dimension since he started teaching in 1951. People used to laugh at him, but now it was a current topic to be discussed. He told me: "*We don't know who wrote the Veda's or the Bible. Nobody knows. Nobody should bother about my name. The aim of this institute is to create a vast movement towards holistic health. We are discussing a new building with a possible modular approach with nature and gardens*". This building was a project that had already mentioned. Dr Basu had also taken considerable interest in the new purpose-built place for health care.

Spirituality: Detachment or Embodiment?

I was aware in the west, both that spirituality had many meanings, and people engaged in a plurality of spiritual health seeking strategies, influenced by cultural therapies throughout the world. Different practices came from different philosophies. For example, shamanic practices of Native American, African and Australian peoples suggested one should be fully embodied on earth. In contrast other traditions, whose influence came from the East suggested we should practise detachment from the body. I asked Dr Basu how he understood embodiment and detachment. He suggested those who engaged in spiritual or esoteric practices, who didn't look after their physical bodies at the same time, may suffer ill health. Then he went on to explain consciousness according to Sri Aurobindo's hierarchical representation, and its relationship to health. He showed us how the physical, social, mental and spiritual dimensions of health could be better understood in relation to different planes of consciousness.

I asked Dr Basu whether Sri Aurobindo considered humans should detach from the body or become more fully embodied. *"This is a very interesting question because in traditional Indian spirituality the words detachment and liberation were always more favoured. Sri Aurobindo favoured the word 'transformation'. Transformation means you have to transfigure. In transfigurement, you do not detach from the body, you detach from the wrong vibrations, and you de-link yourself from the wrong movements. In this way you become a fit instrument for the manifestation of higher principles in your life itself, and not in a distant heaven. You have to concern yourself with the body, you cannot disregard it."*

"Before, in the ascetic tradition, people usually wanted to neglect the body. Ascetic detachment often meant neglecting the body, but here detachment means inner detachment, and a de-linking from the wrong vibrations, for each one of the wrong vibrations can lead to ill health or disease."

He explained that physical illness was the last stage in the manifestation process of an inner disharmony. And once illness had manifested in the human body, it could be slow to heal. He explained how humans could tap into universal energy, and also use the mind to will the body to heal itself. *"It is as if the body has a personality of its own, or a consciousness of its own, which can be developed. The body is like an instrument: the body consciousness can be developed in such a way that a mental will or suggestion can affect it directly."*

Other staff at SAIIIHR explained the relationship between physiological illness and different levels of consciousness. They followed Sri Aurobindo's vision, explaining about different layers of consciousness. They said symptoms people presented with were the tip of the iceberg: *"the physical body is a manifestation of physical consciousness, supported by the vital (emotional) energy level. Behind the vital is the mind, or mental level. These are layers of a being, and the inmost is the soul, which supports everything, without which the physical layer would not be there. When that descends into material consciousness manifestation takes place."*

If staff offered treatments which acted on the physical level, they felt it would work for some time, but would not be deep enough, if the problem was elsewhere. They said for something at the vital level, the energy would need to be corrected before the physical level would stop having the problem. *"If the problem was at the level of the mind, for example a misunderstanding of ideas or concepts, then you could end up with a physical problem which could not be corrected without going to that level."* At a very simple level, this sounds similar to western ways of addressing psycho-somatic symptoms.

Dr Pandey, another psychiatrist with the team also explained the theory of layers of consciousness to me. *"Sri Aurobindo reveals that there are different layers. For me, he was the first mystic who described it so coherently in a language that is comprehensible to use. It becomes so comprehensible to me that there are levels, their meanings, how they influence and affect us, and how we can work upon them. He revealed a whole world. There is so much, even about illness, and the inner view. We have the outer view, the medical and the biological derangement, or the germs. We need to know about the inner view, the subtle forces, and how one can work on them, or be protected from them. All these things are revealed in Sri Aurobindo and the Mother's writings."*

I have included a glossary in the appendix, to define some terms informants used during interviews, with which I was not familiar. I created a list based on the book by Satprem (Adventures of Consciousness) first published in 1968.

Spiritual Approaches to Education

Using a spiritual approach to treat a patient, Dr Pandey said a doctor needed to be aware of inner forces that affect health: he or she should invoke a higher power, and use the concept of faith deliberately. All these elements could be used in addition to the usual care. Such a practitioner, he suggested, would prefer not to use strong drugs and should consider low doses for patients, just enough to allow the body to recover: *"from a spiritual view we would prefer not to use very strong or violent remedies. We would detest the use of many strong analgesics for pain-killers, that lull the consciousness and induce sleep, and other very strong medicines which cause a violent action on physical consciousness. If medicines are used, they should be low doses and not very strong, just to give a little support to the body to recover. We allow the body's healing processes to take over. So medicines are like a stop-gap, for immediate action."*

Dr Pandey was explicit that in emergencies, direct medical action was needed: *"Even in cases of mental distress, if the person has come in a violent state, you give an injection. But to keep putting him on high doses of anti-psychotic or anti-depressant, or immediately giving him ECT, I would not like to do that. I would like to put him on a relatively low dose and start working with him, on his inner life, to the extent that it is possible. In a grossly psychotic or disorganised state, you have got to wait until there is some order. Till then I would like to invoke peace in myself, open my self to grace, which would affect the patient indirectly. Then the patient and the doctor become one unit."* This seemed similar to a mindfulness and compassionate approach[73],[74] of which western trained medical and health care staff were aware.

I had spoken earlier (Chapter 10) to the two lecturers in philosophy about what they would do, if they were in a position to change the curriculum for students. Both said they felt the philosophy curriculum they taught was culture bound and not relevant to the direct experience of their students. They wanted academics to reflect on whether the system limited knowledge according to its own beliefs. I asked the psychiatrist Dr Pandey what he would do, if he could change the curriculum in medical colleges, and could design an additional course for psychiatrists. I asked him what subject areas he would include.

He told me *"The spiritual element is missing, so first of all I would introduce that to students, in our education, at all levels, and medical education is no exception. If you don't introduce that, then the whole sense, direction, and purpose is missing."*

"Medical students, and psychiatrists are no exception, they get carried away by the materialist and the mechanical view of life. The whole thing turns towards commercialisation."

"When I use the word 'spiritual' I should give a note of caution, that we should not confuse it with moral, ethical, religious, or occult teachings, or even philosophy. Spirituality is something to do with the awakening of our own deepest true self. The occult deals with forces and energies of other dimensions. It has some role regarding other energy levels and other vibrations, and should be introduced in its own way."

"Morals and ethics have something to do with our own personal value systems and that is necessary for a physician to know in terms of patient care. Religion is a belief system, which I believe should not be tampered with. So based on an individual belief system, and a person's own background, I would like to introduce the fifth element, the spiritual element which is distinct.

"Students would be taught that two different illnesses can arise from the same psychological source... Then we go to the psychological roots and we help the patient change their attitude and thereby initiate the healing process from within, outwards."

Dr Pandey told me about some key concepts: inner awareness of subtle energies, invoking 'divinity', faith, being aware of the strength of meditation, and allowing the body's own healing process. *"Firstly we need to become aware of the inner disciplines, the forces, at different levels, to be aware of them and work on them. Two, we can invoke a higher power, a higher consciousness. Three, faith is very important to health care. We know about it but we should be more conscious of it, to use it deliberately. We know about the placebo effect. We can use these elements in addition to what we have been doing for care."*

Holism and Homoeopathy

The SAIIIHR practice homoeopaths told me their training for homoeopathy was similar to that of allopathic medicine. Instead of doing chemical pharmacology, they did homoeopathic pharmacology: *"we study all subjects which an allopathic doctor would do, like anatomy, physiology, medicine, surgery. Only the pharmacy part of it is different: allopathy teaches about drugs, whereas we were taught about homoeopathy and the philosophy behind it."*

Dr Pachegoankar, senior homoeopath explained how training in allopathic and homoeopathic medicine was different: with the latter less expensive. He said: *"There is less extensive investigation and machinery required, so homoeopathy is a less expensive technique, both in its education and practice."* He emphasised that with homoeopathy, practitioners did not specialise: the treatment was based on a holistic perspective. *"This means we consider the family background, and grandparents and we study so many generations, and then we devise the treatment on constitutional lines. There was no possibility of having experts specialising within this field. One can be an expert homoeopath, but one would not specialise in one part of the body, for example ophthalmic treatment, ENT, or gynaecology."*

His colleague, Dr Arti worked with her patients using a compassionate counselling framework, and she illustrated how she interacted with her patients. *"There are some doctors who would just ask about physical conditions, and then prescribe based on that. There are some who would look behind the problem, and see why the problems started, and they will try to counsel them. Some without any apparent counselling will try to guide them in such a way then give them medicine and help so that the patient comes out of their particular situation and also recovers physically…"*

She continued: "*whenever a person comes to you, there is a reason why they have come to you. Whenever they come, it is with a different aspect towards life, not one that necessarily matches yours. So when you listen to their problems and when you see a solution... you see that there are no solutions, but something inside you is also working on it, at a subtle level. Often whenever I am interviewing my patient, they may cry because I am touching a sensitive topic... and then they feel relieved after that. During that time, they pour out everything they have in their lives. I am giving a sympathetic ear, as well as interacting. I am not just passively listening to everything. I feel their pain and joy. I am a part of that person for that moment.*"

Holism and Flower Remedies

Spiritual approaches like those mentioned above by Dr Arti, meant practitioners looked deeper than physical symptoms. Another member of staff had originally trained in allopathic medicine, but had also explored homoeopathy, although she felt it had some limitations. She explained: "*I felt people were stuck at a deeper level. For example when I gave a homoeopathic dose, the symptoms would subside, the person would feel better but the problem would still not go, and the person would not glow with complete health. Most often there were patterns that people were repeating. The remedy would work well on a physical or psychological level, but would not help the person completely. I was not completely satisfied.*"

She began looking into flower remedies: "*I thought, what is the water of a flower going to do? Even though I knew that the Mother had given them significances, which touched to the core of the flower. She had understood the inherent vibration in the flower... It is like the remedies are unlocking levels, and connecting you to your source. Then through that connexion, the links with your physical being are built up. They are very subtle. It can only be described as an opening to the light."*

Dr Miovic had also told me about flower essences working on human consciousness, at the level of the soul. Flowers were believed to be the highest and purest form of manifestation, and were used as part of devotional rituals and worship. *"People assume that counselling works only at the mental level, but if counselling is truly effective, then it can change symptoms at a physical level. So the primary remedy might be on the mental level or on the vital level as with homoeopathy; or with flower remedies which act very well at a subtle level, but the mind will also get clear and the physical body will also heal."*

"In a flower, perfection happens spontaneously, though in a human being it could also happen spontaneously".

SUMMARY

The philosophies of health that I'd uncovered through speaking to professionals in Pondicherry seemed to embody holistic spiritual principles. Staff in the medical team at Pondicherry presented the need for balance between detachment from the world, and being embodied and fully of this world. They had mentioned the old divisions between body, mind, and soul, which now needed to be integrated. Many worked within Sri Aurobindo's philosophies of health and his concept of layers of consciousness.

I'd spoken to a former Director General of Health in India, and it seemed as though the seeds sown, so many decades ago, were bearing fruit, and spirituality was now considered an important factor in health. In the UK, the Department of Health had produced a report[75] outlining guidelines for health care practitioners on the importance of religion and faith.

In Pondicherry I had learnt different psychiatrists preferred to modify levels of medication for their patients, so as not to lull their senses. I wondered whether this would be considered as a strategy by psychiatrists in the UK. Would it fit with scientific beliefs about the role of randomised controlled trials with fixed dosage on the efficacy of medication? There seemed to be many subtle ways of understanding health, which went far deeper than I realised, beyond addressing symptoms, emotions, or psychology. It called into question the nature of existential reality and beliefs about the 'self'. In the following chapter I continue by exploring existential paradigms of the body and the self.

Chapter Twelve

EXISTENTIAL PARADIGMS

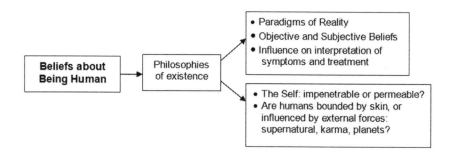

| Beliefs about Being Human | → | Philosophies of existence | → | • Paradigms of Reality
• Objective and Subjective Beliefs
• Influence on interpretation of symptoms and treatment |
| | | | ↘ | • The Self: impenetrable or permeable?
• Are humans bounded by skin, or influenced by external forces: supernatural, karma, planets? |

Influence of Beliefs

Why are our beliefs important? They are important because they influence our theories about the origins of mental ill health and what steps we take towards treatment and healing. In UK beliefs are important because they influence whether or not some members of the population access medical heath care. We human beings hold beliefs that usually fit within particular paradigms. Our beliefs inform our theories of illness causation, our health seeking strategies, and the kinds of treatment we agree to take. Our beliefs help us to understand why we are ill, why now, why us? Our beliefs about existential reality influence how we address our health, and where we place ourselves on earth or within the cosmos.

A paradigm is a model, or pattern of reality. It is a set of assumptions, beliefs, or opinions on how we understand our existence in the world. Scholars have written about paradigm blindness: that is, the inability to see beyond one's own paradigm, which is intrinsic and therefore invisible[76]. There are different models of reality, for example: the earth is flat; the earth is round and at centre of the universe; the sun sets and the moon rises; and the earth is round and rotates. Only one of the above models is considered to be true these days by common consensus, but the others were considered true at earlier times in history. For example in the 15th century we thought Christopher Columbus would sail off the edge of the earth, rather than around it, and 16th century Galileo was put to trial for suggesting the earth revolved around the sun, rather than it being at the centre of the universe.

There are other examples of beliefs, relating to life and health and death: you only live once; you only live once, then die and go to heaven or hell; you are born, live a bit, die, your soul survives then reincarnates; or when you die you turn into an ancestral spirit or a ghost. Our beliefs in these latter statements may depend on the religion we were born into, our country of residence, or any direct experience or direct cognition we may have had in our lives. However, beliefs about different models of reality may be held concurrently by people of the same ethnicity or religion.

There are also different models of belief concerning the human body and how it works. Western understanding assumed our body was bounded by skin, and for a while we assumed that illness occurred when something intruded through an opening, or when the body was damaged by physical trauma. Nowadays, there is wide acceptance of emotional and psychological damage which may influence the well being of body cells. Others believe the human self may be permeable and influenced by external supernatural factors.

Objective and Subjective Beliefs

In the early 20th century some anthropologists may have patronised peoples they studied, and assumed their own beliefs and knowledge were more advanced[77]. Today anthropologists undertaking fieldwork use the terms 'emic' and 'etic': the former to describe concepts from an informant's subjective 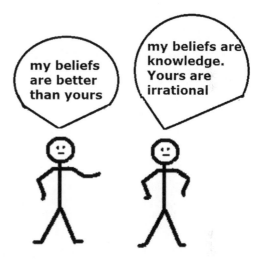 understanding of meaning, and the latter to describe concepts from the investigator's 'objective' understanding. Recently anthropologists developed new subtlety: they were aware of emic explanations and more careful about imposing their own etic interpretations[78].

The two terms address issues around our concern with the nature of objectivity itself. They are particularly relevant when studying mental health and well being, when there may be a wide gap between practitioners trained in western ways, and service users with quite different beliefs about causation and treatment.

There may be a gap between mental health practitioners and service users from the same cultural background, with the former trained in a medical model, and the latter believing in a recovery or a spiritual model. How might we bridge this gap between paradigms and different models of health? Perhaps the best way we can start is by acknowledging a gap exists.

I recently heard about the Ladder of Inference[79], [80]. This describes a technique whereby we (humans) short circuit information, and only perceive the kinds of reality we want. Humans tend to begin with real data and experience, then we select the data we want, give it meaning, develop assumptions, come to conclusions and develop beliefs, which are the basis of our actions, which create additional real data[81]. Using this strategy, we may tend to conduct, authorise or fund research within the boundaries of our own frameworks of knowledge.

The remainder of this chapter offers a summary of existential paradigms presented in earlier parts of the book. It explores beliefs people have about being human, their philosophies of existence and how these influence both the interpretation of their symptoms, and the treatment strategies that they follow. It discusses beliefs about the boundaries of human life, whether humans are only identified within their skins, or whether they are permeable and susceptible to outside influences, like the so called 'supernatural dimensions' of ghosts, ancestors, *djinn*, and the planets. The book explores peoples' beliefs about religion and faith, and the ways devotional rituals, pilgrimage and prayer were said to facilitate healing and mental peace.

Overview of paradigms

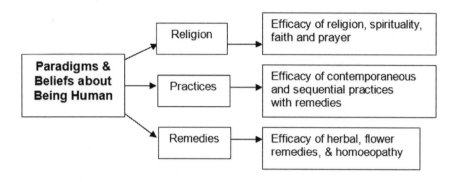

In this section I discuss the different paradigms and healing modalities mentioned in preceding chapters. Earlier chapters have shown people undertake and engage in a synchronistic plurality of strategies for their mental well being. They may go to the doctor, the psychiatrist, traditional and religious healers, clairvoyants or astrologers in a sequential or contemporaneous order. It is normal in India to engage in therapeutic treatments with healers whose practices cover quite different existential paradigms, and different healing modalities.

Continuum of well being and illness

In chapter one, we heard the seer and astrologer SriRam appeared to oscillate between being clairvoyant and psychotic. The psychiatrist either medicated him, or when he was in good mental health used him for his clarity of vision. The psychiatrist, Dr Basu seemed comfortable working within two paradigms: one with the medical models of SriRam presenting symptoms of psychosis which required drugs to treat, and the other with him in good health, as a resource to access subtle realms, to provide additional information about other clients. The doctor also invited a clairvoyant of more mature years to work with him.

Kolkata: medical and religious strategies

In chapter two, there was an interview with a religious cleric (*molovi*) and his healing strategies within the Muslim faith, and we saw the ways he treated his clients with both prayers and amulets. He also discerned who needed to be referred to the psychiatrist for treatment and drugs. The cleric treated his clients for *djinn* and spirit possession, assessed those who he considered required psychiatric help, and referred them on. He also seemed to work within two paradigms: he considered some symptoms required religious or spiritual treatments, and other symptoms were organic and best treated within the bio-medical model of western pharmacology.

The cleric could differentiate between the various symptoms of the clients who visited his home clinic in the village of Jhuruli, on the Bangladesh borders. The clients the *molovi* treated himself were influenced he said, by subtle beings in ethereal space, whereas the psychiatrist used treatments based on substances of the material world. The cleric explained that if Muslim people deviated from Koranic teachings, then this may make them susceptible to occult (hidden) forces. He explained psychiatrists only treated symptoms, while his religious practices treated the cause of symptoms. Both men considered spiritual and religious pursuits and scientific research could co-exist.

Kolkata: contemporaneous treatments

Within chapter three we learnt patients in Kolkata used a variety of treatments both contemporaneously and sequentially. They saw doctors and psychiatrists who worked within the bio-medical model of health, and saw 'traditional healers' who used religious or subtle healing. In the psychiatrist's clinic, we observed that an individual consultation may involve over twenty people being present to support the patient, and this meant the western model of 'individual' healthcare may need to be evaluated differently from a more culturally appropriate perspective. Face to Face consultation was not one to one, as we might understand, but it was consultation with all supporting family and staff. This was often a preferred way among new migrants in UK[82]. In Kolkata, the whole experience of a 'visit to the doctor' was considered part of therapeutic activities, including discussions with other patients and their carers in the waiting room.

Alongside the bio-medical doctors, psychologists and psychiatrists, patients might see: priests; medical herbalists; homoeopaths; traditional healers (*oja*) and teachers (*guru*); astrologers and architectural specialists (*vastusilpi*). Medical herbalists used substances that were found in mundane reality, homoeopathy worked by using an essence of a substance, traditional healers may use occult or supernatural health methods, gurus may use inspirational teachings, astrologers may interpret healing based on the alignment of planets, while *vastusilpi* would consider the effect of spatial relationships on health in a person's home. Again this required a fusion of treatments from different healing modalities and paradigms. Patients and their relatives considered both mundane and supernatural causality of symptoms at the same time.

Patients' symptoms included emotional repression, or suppression; confusion and delusion; violence and self harm; obsession, perversion and meaningless talk. We learnt there were different kinds of tolerance to these symptoms depending on whether one was in an urban or rural setting. The alternation of swinging between a gifted state and a psychiatric state was common, as was moving between supernatural gifted skills and mundane psychotic behaviour, in the same person. Some patients seemed to be on a continuum, balancing between wellness in the mundane world of religious practice, and tipping into psychosis and over sensitivity to the subtle realms. Temples such as the one in Tirol, West Bengal were used by patients for both religious prayer and occult rituals and practices.

The psychiatrist Dr Basu himself moved between the boundaries of different paradigms, being trained in western psychiatry and pharmacology, however he also followed philosophies of the sage Sri Aurobindo and acknowledged divine aspects of consciousness. Working with patients he diagnosed a range of mundane, spiritual or supernatural causes for symptoms, and suggested treatment strategies that were appropriate to each type of causation. Patients felt this was a realistic way to address their needs, which covered all the options to tackle suffering and distress. For example one young man mentioned earlier was attacked by *djinn*, had financial problems and became extremely violent. He was given Koranic amulets by the Muslim cleric, and carried chained on a bicycle rickshaw to the psychiatrist, who diagnosed him with bipolar disorder, gave him an injection to calm him down, and then lithium tablets.

The case studies mentioned earlier illustrate that the psychiatrist considered both medical and occult (hidden) theories of illness causation and suggested therapeutic strategies that took each into consideration. For example a young woman who was repeatedly suicidal was given maintenance drugs between episodes, and Dr Basu suggested she undertake prayer rituals and burn camphor. Another patient said she had visited both Hindu and Muslim healers, at the same time as having consultations with the psychiatrist. The psychiatrist offered western pharmacology to one young man who was in a locked nursing home, and he crossed paradigm boundaries by suggesting past life therapy might throw light on his case. Another man, also in the locked nursing home appeared desperate to kill himself. The psychiatrist put him under 24 hour observation, and decided to give him ECT treatment. He also suggested the patient's brothers say prayers for the dead, which would help lift any discarnate entities that were with him, in case he had picked up spirits of individuals who had committed suicide near his home.

It was normal for both psychiatrist and patients to consider plural theories of causation that crossed different paradigms of existence. The underlying assumption was that the distress, however severe, was an episode, which could be recovered from, and 'normal' life resumed. This can be compared to beliefs about the 'recovery movement' held first by service users in UK, and now taken on by service providers[83].

Theories of illness causation

In chapter 4, the causal factors which patients said triggered their illness also belonged within several paradigms: social and relationship explanations (e.g. poor treatment by in-laws, desertion, witnessing a traumatic death, repressed emotions, and bereavement) and the supernatural (presence of a deceased relative, hallucinations). If people witnessed a suicide or an unnatural death, they said it affected their mental well being. One key problem married women expressed was due to patrilocal residence (living within their husband's extended family) and being harshly treated. This was exacerbated if they failed to conceive early. Men also had theories of causation which crossed paradigm boundaries. They included social and emotional reasons like loss or bereavement, or quarrelling with the family, financial problems, or substance abuse. Also there were occult triggers for mental distress: over use of occult rituals and clairvoyance; being attacked by *djinn*; and failure to recharge a religious protective charm.

Practitioners gave examples of causal factors for triggers to mental distress which covered different paradigms: biological; psychological; environmental; planetary alignments; karma; and spirit possession. In chart no.5.2 the pharmacological treatments used by patients are given in one column, and the alternative treatments in the following column. Dr Basu explained he considered diagnosis on different levels, being aware of a patient's inner being, levels of consciousness, their soul and spirit, and then he modified their medication accordingly. He was aware some of the diagnoses he gave his patients did *"not fit into classical ICD10 and DSM IV"*. He preferred a holistic approach to diagnosis.

Religious and Spiritual Treatments

The fieldwork indicated temples, churches and mosques were used throughout India for alleviating mental distress, through pilgrimage and performing prayer rituals. Prayer and religious rituals propitiating deities were also considered an important part of treatment strategies, which were done at the same time as taking pharmacology to alleviate symptoms. Patients believed the religious aspects addressed the wider causes of mental distress, while the drugs addressed the symptoms. Pilgrimages to temples like Suryanarkoil (for the nine planets) addressed the astrological causes of mental distress, while the wearing of amulets supported the healing process. At temples and mosques attendants used rituals to cleanse attendees of impurities and shock away discarnate entities. This meant being 'brushed' at one mosque in Nagore and being sharply 'flicked' and anointed with holy water at a temple in Gunasilam, or being fanned with smoking incense at Rameshwaram. Bathing also eased mental well being, either in religious water tanks, beside wells, or in the sea.

In a couple of temples in Tamil Nadu, I saw places where the mentally ill were restrained, or housed in closed off areas. The underlying assumption was that they would be able to take up the healing vibration at those religious places and become cured of their mental distress. (After the year 2000, chaining stopped, except in the constant presence of a relative). Those who were restrained in or near temple complexes had daily routines which involved a perambulation around the walkways of the shrines to take up the healing vibrations. Dr Basu felt it might be possible to incorporate the taking of pharmaceuticals at the same time as being housed at a temple complex. He wanted to develop a sacred healing site to incorporate religious rituals and supplement patients with medical drugs and healing. This would integrate the boundaries between paradigms and employ the best strategies of each.

People of any faith went to all manner of religious organisations. Their beliefs stretched beyond religious affiliation, and they often regarded a mosque or a church as having stronger power to heal them. Physical evidence was provided of cure and change, for example in one mosque, iron and glass objects were said to have been coughed up by patients as part of their cure. These physical artefacts were exhibited to provide evidence that occult or religious healing strategies worked. It seemed normal for paradigms to fuse together in this way.

How does this fit within western models of mental health and psychiatry? The mental health 'survivor' movement has become more and more vocal in their dissatisfaction with western models of psychiatry and health care[84]. They felt the bio-medical model was inadequate for addressing their health needs: they described themselves as 'survivors' of the psychiatric system[85]. However, some medical professionals in UK were very uncomfortable with the term 'survivor', and felt it should only be used by those who had experienced holocaust or genocide, rather than by those who had been within the care of a psychiatric system. Further insight into the survivor perspective can be found in the Mental Health Testimony Archive, a collaborative project with Mental Health Media and the British Library, which held 50 video interviews with mental health service users, who had

had first-hand knowledge of psychiatric asylums[86]. The Citizens Commission on Human Rights prepared a Compendium setting out their perspectives on psychiatry, calling it a 'destructive force'.[87] Through these challenging and contrasting views, there may be valuable principles to learn.

In India it was normal to consider mental distress and mental peace together, as they were part of a continuum, and religious and spiritual places were used both to maintain mental peace and alleviate distress. Rituals and practices that seemed to cross the paradigm divide were included in visits to three temples and one cathedral. The prayer rituals were part of devotional activities in the temples and in front of deities, where pilgrims aspired to have '*darshan*' or catch the eye of the deity. Also there were the soothsayer palm leaf oracles at Vaitheeswarankoil, which were interpreted by specialist families, for those customers who wanted to understand their present and see their future. How do these concepts fit within a western materialist present, where the future is unknown in the future, and the underlying assumption is that it cannot be viewed in the present?

The temple of Suryanarkoil was the place where pilgrims expressed devotion to the planets in order to achieve a peaceful state of mind. In India, the full and dark moon seemed to influence Dr Basu's patients' state of mind. Would any UK psychiatrist claim the moon or planets affected their patients' well being? In towns like Harrow (NW London) where I live, many of the population are Asian from India and Africa, and have commensurate beliefs about the influence of planets on mental health. It was explained to me that planet deities were anthropomorphised like an icon, which carried the vibration of the planet, and were easier to offer devotion to than the planets themselves more directly. Dr Loganathan the medical herbalist had said: *'grass roots people better understand the worship of religious icons, rather than planets'.*

In Rameshwaram bereaved families visited the shore in groups as a memorial to honour their deceased kin. It was a place for ceremonies for mental peace of the living. The ashes of the cremated deceased were rolled in with rice to form balls, representing the deceased, and then left for crows and cows to consume. Cremation was done, together with appropriate prayers to allow the soul to release from the body, so it didn't remain on earth. There is an increasing literature on the efficacy of prayer for well being and healing[88]. In UK some relatives of Asian deceased people cast their ashes into the River Thames.

Other rituals in India included the visiting of shrines, and undertaking religious ablution in the wells of Rameshwaram temple, where the waters were said to ward off sin and insanity. However, in some shrines around Rameshwaram I felt rituals were conducted for tourists in a rather perfunctory manner with a reduced religiosity. At Vailankanni cathedral ("the Lourdes of the Orient") there were votive offerings in the form of body parts in wax, which were offered to Our Lady for healing. The museum by the cathedral exhibited thousands of offerings, given once people had achieved a cure, through divine intervention. Some written thanks were for those who had been spontaneously cured, and therefore did not need 'invasive medicine'. The votive offerings served to carry the pain or distress away from the sick person, and allowed it through prayer and ritual, to be transmuted into wellness.

There was one thing in common at sacred places: whether the presiding deity was Hindu, Muslim or Christian, pilgrims who used these places were from any faith. Once a place had a reputation for divine efficacy, pilgrims of any religion visited it. The location was in the material realm, but the effect of being there and performing rituals was sacred or divine, again crossing boundaries. Prayer in any faith, in any language was considered effective.

The two ashrams I visited, which attracted devotees seeking mental peace, were Sri Ramana Maharshi's in Tiruvanamalai, and Sri Aurobindo's at Pondicherry. Both ashrams had followers from Indian and Western countries of origin. The gurus or sages might be compared to great monks or nuns in UK, whose teachings were respected. Food was prepared by those who resided at these places, and offered in huge communal dining rooms. They might be compared with Christian Retreat Centres in UK, for example like at Douai Abbey inhabited by Benedictine monks, or the secluded Kairos Centre, where visitors might be of any faith and yet request spiritual direction. Alternatively there were secular yet spiritual retreats in UK, like Gaunts House or Hazelwood House.

At Sri Aurobindo's ashram, devotees said there was an energy or a force there that had been brought down to earth by Sri Aurobindo and the Mother. Sri Aurobindo called it a supramental consciousness. In contrast, followers of Sri Ramana Maharshi considered that the divine force was already extant on earth. Sri Ramana Maharshi taught in silence about realisation, insight, and surrender, to be one self, wherever one was, in whatever environment.

The place I stayed at the longest and from where I began and ended my travels was Pondicherry, staying at ashram hotels or residences. I did have some 'paranormal' experiences there, which seemed normal for that place, in that ashram, with those people. Even the psychiatrist had visions. Common consensus was that visions were normal. It was normal for the Mother Mirra Alfassa to have visionary experiences. The paradigm there was that 'extraordinary' or spiritual experiences were normal.

The aim of some people attending the ashram was to manifest those visions, so they benefited practical mundane human life. Sri Aurobindo himself had inspirational insights, was a prolific writer, and the ashram was set up to support people undertaking inner reflection to solve the practical problems of human existence. The ideal was to achieve divine life on earth as part of physical existence. Sometimes it felt to me as if in India philosophers and gurus became so venerated, that their followers expressed devotion towards them.

Treatment Remedies

This section considers treatments and remedies (material substances) which crossed paradigm boundaries, and whose healing modalities worked in different ways. For example: allopathic drugs used pharmacologically active ingredients; herbal remedies used natural pharmacology; homoeopathy treated like with like; acupuncture worked with energy flows; and flower remedies treated conditions with their antidote.

The allopathic pharmacological drugs used by the psychiatrists were generated by those working with biomedical models of health. They were said to act directly with/on disease pathology, as did herbal remedies, which were derived from physical medicinal compounds of plants. However, homoeopathic remedies worked differently to enhance the patient's own healing ability. They were said to stimulate a patient's own healing force, which then eradicated disease, as part of a longer term strategy. However, if a patient urgently needed medication, then homoeopaths worked together with allopathic doctors to address symptoms quickly. The healing mechanism of homoeopathy was like a vaccine, a toxin that had a 'negative vibration' at subtle levels, which could be used by a person, who in time developed a tolerance and overcome it.

Homoeopathic physicians claimed to treat the whole person and not just the parts, by working with subtle energy. Dr Mistry had said earlier: *"Allopathy does not deal with the spiritual level: it is at the extreme edge of the spectrum of physicality*". He explained that allopathy offered only one kind of treatment, which "*does not have a total overview that integrates the mind and emotional feeling at their depths, and all the structures and cells at their depths.*" He explained that western pharmacology dealt with physical illness, but not with subtle energy and consciousness. Homoeopathy was a form of information and intelligence. He suggested for mental health, one had to first exclude organic causes or traumas, and then address spiritual or metaphysical causes. He suggested health care providers became aware of the limits of each of type of remedy, and worked with other therapists to maximise patient benefit.

Although herbal remedies were derived from active pharmacological compounds of plants, some medical herbalists were aware of influences beyond a materialistic paradigm. For example I was told remedies selected from certain plants were modified by the influence and position of planets when the patient was born. Also the plants themselves were said to modify the effect of planetary influence on a person. Plants and trees may themselves be offered as part of devotional rituals, or worship may take place in proximity to them. In diagnosing a person's problems, a medical herbalist would consider both their horoscope and their mundane living environment.

The original knowledge obtained about a plant's medical properties was said to be gleaned through a practitioner tuning their perception into the plant and sensing its properties. Shamans and psychics might do something similar today to find out information, by going into a light trance, or altered state of consciousness. The medical herbalist suggested traditional knowledge on herbal pharmacology could be clinically tested, to support the evidence base. However, he felt it was important to consider the complete range of causations for each patient, before selecting appropriate plant remedies.

Medical herbalists believed mental illness could be caused by karma (the past deeds of a patient's own or their forefathers), and this could be addressed and completed with one particular generation of a family. Some treatment strategies might include making a pilgrimage around appropriate temples. The causality of planetary position and effects of karma were considered as having distant or remote or no causality, by psychiatric practitioners in the west. Theories of causality for mental ill health in UK appeared to be culturally determined, as did treatment. Practitioners in India used information from a combination of paradigms to support their diagnosis and treatment of a patient.

An American psychiatrist visiting Pondicherry used a range of remedies from different paradigms with his patients in the USA. He used established pharmacology with patients who were in a severe psychotic or manic state for scientific and legal reasons, but for some outpatients with chronic depression or anxiety, he suggested they use flower essences. Also, when he worked in a cancer clinic, he said flower essences did not conflict with a patient's chemotherapy or radiation treatment. They worked with the human soul, the psychic being (the psychic was the nucleus of divine consciousness). He suggested a flower's 'vibration' helped support psychotherapy when dealing with emotional issues. Flower essences healed within the consciousness paradigm.

Dr Edward Bach was a medical doctor who conducted research into positive essences that could be used to heal a person, and he found tinctures made from flowers were a most positive remedy. Instead of making remedies using homoeopathic methods he discovered they were more effective when made using sun potentisation. I was told psychotherapy used together with flower remedies would work at a deep emotional level. Flower remedies were useful because they did not interact with allopathic drugs, in the way that the active pharmacology of herbal medicine did, and they did not have side effects.

I wonder how psychiatrists and psychologists in UK would respond to these alternative treatments. Some are already considering alternative healing strategies, but others remain silent. I wonder how many would ask about our spiritual lives (though I did have a GP, now retired, who offered Christian prayer for ill health.)

Explanatory models

Explanatory models for ill health came within a variety of paradigms: materialist, psychological, subtle energy, and consciousness. Part Three set out peoples' explanatory models for mental ill health, and these included mundane theories of illness causation (chapter 8) and esoteric theories of illness causation (chapter 9). When I interviewed people inevitably mundane explanations were mentioned first, like: substance abuse, physiological disorders and psychological responses to events, environmental factors, and the effects of disequilibrium.

The last one: 'disequilibrium' was said to be the result of causes which bridged boundaries between mundane and esoteric influences. It included the effects of karma, planetary alignment, angry deities, the unsettled dead (like ghosts), as well as a lack of balance between mind, body and emotions. Dr Basu claimed harmonious therapy would address these different levels of dissonance. He felt a mismatch could occur if a person over-used the spiritual aspects of their inner being, but didn't take care of their physical health.

When I began my career as an ethnographer and conducted fieldwork abroad, I acknowledge that I may not have recorded everything I observed, as some events did not fit within the parameters of my research plan. I would like to suggest there may be other researchers or observers whose cultural beliefs may have influenced the kinds of data they recorded. This issue is particularly important when conducting research into mental health promotion strategies in a multicultural society like Britain. It is relevant to consider Indian explanatory models for mental distress, because many Asian peoples are resident in UK. In the London Borough of Harrow where I worked, some wards had 64% black and Asian residents. According to the 2011 census, almost a third of Harrow's population were Asian. It is my opinion that if front line health care professionals in UK were empathetic towards the beliefs of others, then they may be considered as being more helpful by their clients[89]. In 2014 Professor Anil Jain in Manchester[90] suggested a new approach for those who practice medicine and health care with UK populations: that ongoing 'cultural humility' be practiced rather than cultural competence.

In India, the esoteric factors believed to trigger mental distress were numerous, and in UK our choices today are: to accept them as culturally normal, or as culturally delusional (depending where our own beliefs about reality lie). Beliefs include those mentioned above: planetary influences, karma, reincarnation, effects of subtle energies, and spirit possession. There was also a belief that occult practices, which were not supervised by specialists, could result in symptoms of mental distress. Furthermore, there were explanations attributed to reincarnation: for example, visitors to a home where children had learning disabilities explained they were born like that because this was their first incarnation as humans, from being animals in previous lives. In the UK service providers and their clients do not need to hold the same belief systems, but it may help communication and healing to suspend judgement, and acknowledge and discuss both sets of beliefs, and arrive at a negotiated treatment strategy.

❖❖❖

The Human Self

In this section my intention is to explore beliefs about the nature of human existence; theories about the nature of reality; and beliefs about subtle levels of existence. I set out concepts of self and expanded self in relation to theories of illness causation. I also present different cultural understandings of the self: the boundaried and limited individual self of western psychology; and the extended family and social 'sense of self' found in Asian and African societies.

I had interviewed several people who made comments about the 'self', and explained their understanding of self within caste and community. They gave examples of the term 'outcaste' and some spoke about how meaningless the term 'caste' was for them. My intention was to unpack what interviewees understood by: the individual self, the social self, personal identity, caste identity, the psychic self, and the soul. I wanted to gain insight into the complexity and subtlety of meanings.

It seemed people I spoke to in India thought the self could expand as well as extend, so it developed faculties for remote sensing, perceiving the future; or their self felt infiltrated by other beings, which were not human. I set out interviewee's core existential beliefs on culture and spiritual explanatory models for mental ill health. I presented paradigms of different ways of thinking, and invited the philosophers and psychiatrists to envision what changes they might make, to university curricula, if they had they authority to incorporate more spiritual or more culturally appropriate course modules. In chapter 11, I asked one psychiatrist how he would address his concerns about training in mental health, if he was in a position to modify the curriculum.

The Self: Extended and Expanded

In the west, it was assumed that 'I' meant the individual person, bounded by the skin, the surface of which formed an edge, beyond which the outer world existed. This was the individual 'I', the self, or the conscious person. However, this was not the case with members of ethnic minority groups in UK[91]. Dr Basu explained that the 'Indian individual self' did not carry the same meaning as a 'British individual self'. The Indian self incorporated the extended family, and the residential community. He believed the typical Indian 'self' was an 'extended self', unlike the 'individual western self'. For this reason he considered individual counselling or psychotherapy with a patient would not be fully beneficial unless supplemented with family therapy. He believed socio-cultural intervention by trained social workers was necessary, as was contacting support systems in the community. Support of extended family members, friends, spiritual groups, and occult support systems was needed.

This perspective was also held by Asian and African migrants, refugees and asylum seekers in the UK, who considered it normal for their extended family to be involved in individual consultations. Migrant populations like the Gujarati and Somali in UK also wanted holistic family support and involvement[92]. This strong feeling came from populations which had become dis-embedded from their territories and places of origin, either by choice or by force. Some UK citizens from minority ethnic groups felt that 'self' or 'kinship' extended to people of the same gender, colour, or religion.

Dr Basu continued and he emphasised that in India the outer self extended to a person's social and kin network. He said: *"Insecurity in any point of the extended self affects a person's well-being. Here in India, 'I' means my friends, my family members, and even my goddess*

Kali who I worship, as the main deity in my house. The meaning 'I' is very extended in India. When somebody comes to me from a joint family in a village, even if he has lived alone in the city for 20 years, if I give him a form to fill out, which asks whether he is living in a joint, extended family or single, he will tick joint. He will not tick that he is living as single, because he identifies himself with the joint family in the village. He will consider his condition in the city as temporary, even after 20 years. In India this outer self is an extended social self, where we include everybody plus the main house deity."

Caste, Religious Affiliation, and Place

Although some western academics believed the concept of caste important, it was clear among *ashramites* at Pondicherry, that caste identity was not considered significant. However, elsewhere in India other people thought caste was extremely important as an identifier of self. I've included interviews with two people to highlight differences regarding this point.

In-caste. In Solapur, when I was introduced to Professor Katkar (lecturer in philosophy), I asked him about the way in which caste situated a person within society. He explained his full identifying details, of caste, place of origin, and sub-caste which located him socially and geographically when he met another person.

He chanted: "I *am Hindu, brahmin. Among brahmins in this Maharashtra area, there are sub-castes: I am nayshasta. Then there is a sub-community: kahari, I belong to the deshasta brahmin community".*

"In our community each brahmin family has a connexion with certain texts (Vedas), and we belong to rigved. Each ved has its own branch, and we belong to the sharkara branch. And each brahmin family is connected to a particular scriptural treatise, which prescribes certain rituals connected with 'soma' sacrifice. These are traditionally known as kalpa sutra, and ours is ashpulai kalpi sutra".

"So I am a Hindu Brahmin, belonging to *rigved*, the *shankara* branch of *rigved*, with which is affiliated the *ashpulai kalpa sutra*. This is my traditional identity. If a saint, a yogi, or a spiritual preceptor, if he comes before me, and I prostrate before him, this is what I say".

"Then we have gotras, we are born in a family lineage, which reaches back to some vedic sage, whom is the origin of our particular family, and their name is degotrani. I'd belong to jaabenadegotr." He chanted his identity again, and then laughed, for it went on for so long. Included in his identity was the fact that his family came from a village called Kaatih, near Solapur. *"Because the family was in Kaatih, so we are called Kaatika, Or Katkar. So we are situated with a very precise identity."* Professor Katkar indicated how much his identity was in relationship to his family lineage, his religious community, scriptural texts, and his place of origin. As an individual person he was clearly situated in the world. However, in Pondicherry, among the members of the Sri Aurobindo ashram, people perceived less or no need for using caste as their personal identifier.

Outcaste: Dr Bisht came to Pondicherry from Darhwal in the Himalayan mountains from the state of Utaranchal. It was he who had originally suggested to the World Health Organisation they needed to consider the topic of spirituality and health. He told me in his opinion the topic of caste was a preoccupation of western academics. I had heard this point of view expressed before by other members of the medical team.

Dr Bisht explained about his family: *"My official religion is Hindu, and my official caste is Kshatriya, but I do not believe in any of this. My grandfather was in the British army in Burma, and my father was the field postmaster for Anglo American forces in Manila and Japan, and the Far East. My family was out-casted in my grandfather's time, 100 years ago. This was because we did not believe in caste in the village, and so we were out caste. My grandfather was a staunch Arayasamajist, a group established by Dyananda Saraswathi, who didn't believe in caste. All my family were soldiers, some with the forces in Lahore."*

"These days in that village, nobody worries what caste you belong to. But you know, when you are out caste, in order to come back, you are supposed to go to the river Ganges, shave your head, take a dip, and then you become purified. Till then nobody will speak or smoke with you, nobody will eat rice with you. It happened to my grandfather's family."

Beyond Caste: I asked another member of the Medical Team about caste. This was the psychiatrist Dr Pandey, and my question elicited a similar response. *"From the traditional caste point of view, I belong to the Brahmin caste, but then, in Sri Aurobindo's yoga, all these distinctions get blurred. So from a spiritual point of view, I really don't know what my caste is, except for by birth."*

Likewise another ashramite, Mr Sircar, who was originally born to Kaiyastu parents of the Hindu religion. On the subject of caste, he said, *"We don't believe in such things. They are warriors but those things have vanished nowadays, and we don't follow the caste system."* He continued: *"also I never believed in gods and goddesses, and I hated the hypocrisy of the so-called religion."*

Caste had been an identifier of a person's occupation, religious affiliation and geographical location, and still was throughout India. However, in Pondicherry, those who followed the philosophy of Sri Aurobindo and the Mother had chosen to release their attachment to indicators of their origins. In the next part I look at concepts and faculties of the incarnate self and the physical being.

Subtle Levels of Existence

Beliefs about the incarnate self were complex, especially those beliefs about self that went beyond the physical incarnate human person embodied on earth. Some informants believed there were other beings, which were not in body, but might be embodied, and might influence a living individual's self. Perhaps the closest catch-all translation in English might be the terms 'spirit' or 'ghost' (a person who had lived and died, but not left the earth's 'atmosphere'). The religious studies scholar Graham Harvey has given us an elaborate discussion of 'Other Than Human Beings[93]': the introduction to his book was a most extensive balanced presentation.

In India spiritism (the belief that the dead interact with the living) was often part of cultural explanations for mental distress, and because of this I had asked various people I interviewed about discarnate beings. People referred to different kinds of 'beings', and different elements of a human being: the vital being, psychic being, soul, and disembodied beings (a glossary of Sri Aurobindo's terms are included in Appendix A). In Part Two I described specialist healers at temples and mosques, who worked independently as astrologers, and used subtle levels of healing. In chapter 9 various informants gave examples of how they considered disembodied beings were created, and how they thought they were involved in spirit possession.

Interviews with people in India suggested that there were different models of reality. There were quite different ways of looking at the world: different ways of considering human existence, and subsequently different ways of treating people with mental health problems. It is my opinion that many of us have our own personal bias, our own personal perceptions about human existence, which we may feel strongly about, especially if anyone brushes up against our beliefs. When other peoples' theories of existence are dissonant with our own, we may find it rather challenging, as these kinds of beliefs are core to our very presence on earth. The psychiatrist Kübler-Ross[94] explained five stages of grief: anger, denial, depression, bargaining, and acceptance. These stages may also occur when another person's beliefs come into conflict with our belief systems.

Paradigm shifts

I had a question for Dr Basu, who had written a book on Integral Health[95], and mentioned consciousness and its relationship to health and well being. I asked him to explain what he meant by the relationship between science and spirituality. He said: *"At a certain point of time, a physician understands the reality of life, in a better way than other professionals do because face to face with life and death he can understand his own limitations. In the history of consciousness, a point has come now where things which were hidden before, which were questions which were never raised, things in consciousness which never came on the surface, they are now coming."*

"You see even Freud talked about the repression of the unconscious. Today nobody now represses anything. Everything is now exposed, and you can't explain neurosis any longer by repression. This is a thing which has happened in the history of consciousness which has never happened before. The whole unconscious, the whole subconscious, they are opening up, and they are throwing up many things. It was never so much on the surface, it was always hidden. So consciousness has its own history."

"At this point of time, when everything has become visible, and is opening layers and breaking, we are finding that the borderline between science and spirituality, science and mysticism is also becoming clearer. This also holds within quantum physics as well as in mathematics, so naturally it will be in psychology, and the strict divisions between a psychologist and an occultist, that has to break. Because if psychology is to concern itself with the human mind, then I cannot ignore either the mind of the scientist nor the mind of the mystic. Because I am working with mind, both minds are important."

The point about the role of the practitioner being part of the framework for healing was important, as was the nature of mindfulness. I consulted Dr Pandey who felt the whole paradigm around medicine, psychiatry and health needed to change. He considered medicine needed to take account of the subtle triggers of mental distress. *"There is too much stress on the mechanistic model. I think the paradigm has to change to a consciousness perspective, to the understanding that there is a non-material reality of consciousness, which is primary and fundamental, that the body and all other phenomena are an outgrowth. They are not the cause of consciousness but the result of consciousness. As is the level of consciousness, so is the illness, and so is the cure."*

"The whole paradigm has to change, and only then can we possibly make headway. Right now even when we admit the spiritual element as in W.H.O.'s definition, it is more like lip-service. The spiritual thought should be primary as well as the spiritual concept, and the rest should be seen from there."

I turned towards another psychiatrist Dr Michael Miovic, who worked in Harvard but regularly visited Pondicherry, and asked what studies he had published that were acceptable to the wider community with their need for evidence based medicine. He said: *"I have published some material in NAMAH[96], and I am working on some case studies. I am starting with a paper on the theory of psychology. At a theoretical level, if these things work, the first question is: how on earth could a placebo work? If it works, it pushes the issue of a spiritual reality right to the forefront. And there is really no other way of understanding how an essence could work, other than mere suggestion, without using a metaphysics that is spiritual[97]."*

"I've been working very hard over the last year, on introducing a spiritual framework for psychology into mainstream psychotherapy. It turns out that you can introduce Sri Aurobindo's ideas into mainstream, and you don't need to refer to transpersonal psychology. He stands in his own right. You can introduce Sri Aurobindo into western psychology and his work will stand in its own right".

I hadn't understood clearly and I asked Michael to explain again about the relationship between Sri Aurobindo and Transpersonal Psychology. *"Transpersonal psychology is still confused. You need Sri Aurobindo in order to understand it, but not the other way round. You need him to clarify some of the fuzzy issues of transpersonal psychology, because they don't know what the difference is between the psychic being and the self, and the psychic being and the pranic being".*

"There's a lot of things in yoga psychology that are very well defined, based on thousands of years of experience, that transpersonal psychology does not know about. But the most important concept for practical purposes is Mother's concept of the psychic being. She makes it so simple, and so direct, and relevant to the problems of daily life."

Michael had published a lengthy essay on the topic of non-local mind and consciousness in NAMAH. He had eloquently reviewed experimental and case-based evidence from Western scientific research that supported the claim that consciousness was non-local[98]. The physician Larry Dossey made similar statements about non-local mind: *"I am convinced, that medical science not only has not had the last word, it has hardly had the first word on how the world works, especially when the mind is involved[99]."*

Visions for the Future

In Pondicherry there were clinics that dealt with mental health, where social workers attended patients, there was also a psychiatric hospital on the outskirts of town; and there was a psychiatric ward in Jipmeh hospital. Ashram staff commented that they all used western style medicine, and not 'natural' or 'Indian' treatments. There were only a few doctors who worked integrally both within and outside western medicine using a spiritual approach, and these were people I had interviewed as part of the study.

Dr Loganathan, the medical herbalist had told me about the need for a specific kind of architecture that would help people with mental health problems. "If we use the *traditional medical health care, there is no separation of the mind and body in understanding illness and its treatment. As far as the modern system of medicine is concerned, we are treating only the body, and to the mind and spirit there is more philosophically to be worked out. One may not need any kind of medicine, but one may need the proper design of the room, house, village or land, and the proper colour that suits the mind, that can calm and bring peace to the mind."*

Dr Basu agreed and explained old mental institutions in India were built in the pattern of jails, with a central watch tower, and rooms radiating outwards. He said SAIIIHR was planning a more developed place for an institution, a healing centre of a suitable architectural design, for those with mental health problems, where there were gardens. He told me: *"There needs to be a space for meditating on the essence of being, on the soul. The designs needed to be specific to a rehabilitation centre, where there would be trees and gardens, and space for occupational therapy and artistry. Each space should manifest consciousness, ananda and bliss, and one should manifest knowledge".*

SUMMARY

The style of medicine in India has been mentioned, and the buildings in which it takes place, but what about the paradigm differences? What about the different concepts of 'self' and individual; the concepts of expanded self, and non-local mind; the beliefs in subtle energies and entities; beliefs in disembodied beings and spirit possession; the plurality of treatment options that exist within different healing modalities.

How do we start to acknowledge all of that within western health care, and negotiate and manifest appropriate treatment strategies for patients? I do not have the answers of how we communicate these things both as core subjects within training institutions, nor for post registration staff. However, in the final part, I present the current situation in UK for mental health promotion with minority ethnic groups, and explore what has been done to address the topic of cultural diversity. In the last chapter I make recommendations for a way forward in education and trainng.

PART FIVE

TRANSFERABLE MODELS

Chapter Thirteen

RELEVANCE FOR UK POPULATIONS

Overview

This chapter explores the relevance of mental health practices in India to UK populations. Does the reader think interviews in this book on **'Spiritual Psychiatries,'** are simply a collection of anecdotal narratives generated from specific places in Kolkata and Tamil Nadu in India, or might they be of relevance to people in the UK? I wondered to what extent information and philosophies of health contained within these pages, might be transferable to UK populations.

In the first part I identify concerns that occurred in the 'interim years' in UK, after the DRE (Delivering Race Equality) programme ended, and before the new Equalities Act really took effect. This was a period of time when for a few years, culture and ethnicity seemed to be ignored. I present some initiatives with Black and Asian Minority Ethnic groups (BAME) on mental health promotion, and consider government strategies of that time to address mental health.

New migrants and refugees have particular concerns regarding mental well being[100]. In the last few years (2009 to 2014) various UK government strategies were undertaken to address BAME[101] mental health, and I have commented on a selection of meetings I attended. In 2013 the topic of BAME ethnicity and belief was returning for consideration and discussion, but I wondered to what extent this was being addressed by the new Clinical Commissioning Groups.

The second section addresses issues around Eurocentrism and cultural paradigms. It considers assumptions which were made around the topic of cultural diversity (rather than supporting the development of cultural humility). It examines paradigm problems, raising questions on ways change might be supported or initiated to incorporate the principles of cultural and spiritual paradigms addressed in Part Four of this book. I explore the assumption in UK that the dominant model of health (bio-medicine) was the only model of health. I set out different cultural models of human existence which may result in paradigm problems. I note various models of reality and health which co-exist, but which don't inter-relate, unless cultural humility is put in place to support negotiation.

The third section addresses the population demography in UK cities, which is already suggestive of a need for awareness about cultural models of health. In the capital London the population is ethnically diverse with over eight million people: 40% are from minority ethnic groups, with 32% born outside UK. In the London borough of Harrow 28% are of Indian origin[102]; in Tower Hamlets 20% are of Bangladeshi origin[103]. Using the London borough of Harrow as a case study I present former mental health promotion strategies both voluntary and statutory: from community health groups and Time to Change initiatives, as well as research done for NHS Harrow and the Kings Fund.

The forth section looks at issues around communication and collaboration.

The final chapter explored the ways in which the principles of mental health care were transferable to a more global western market. In addition, a series of educational training options for front line practitioners was put forward, with notes on the UK government response to cultural competency for schools. [Since 2012 schools have had OSTED[104] inspections on SMSC (Spiritual, Moral, Social and Cultural Well Being), but this level of interest has not yet extended to clinical health care.] In the USA cultural competencies are a core part of medical and health care education, whereas in UK the topic is an optional part of the educational curriculum.

Section One: The Interim Years

Good Intentions: Mental Healthcare in UK

Let us start by exploring the recent situation regarding mental health, culture and health care in Britain. I give a brief overview of the Parekh Report, the Care Quality Commission and the Count Me In Census, the DRE Programme (Delivering Race Equality), the Equalities Act, and the Department of Health's Mental Health Strategy. I wanted to explore how these projects influenced government policy on mental health care. Then I present examples of attitudes about mental health and culture I observed in recent conferences and meetings.

The Parekh report, set up by Runnymede Trust in 1998, had a remit to analyse multi ethnic Britain and suggest ways of addressing racial disadvantage and discrimination. One of their recommendations was that professionals employed in health and social services be trained in cultural awareness. They felt these front-line workers had the potential to transform the health care experience of ethnic minority communities. Front-line staff were considered to be key in determining the nature of equality and diversity for service users and staff within an organisation.

Parekh expected medical and health care professionals to maintain a high standard of education and practice self regulation. In the UK there had been government commitments regarding training of professional staff, to address principles of discrimination and cultural competency. However there remained an awareness some practitioners were not adequately trained in cultural literacy and did not always respond appropriately to ethnic diversity issues in their field of work. A five year action plan was initiated in 2005, on Delivering Race Equality in the field of mental health. Community development workers were trained and deployed in health, but by 2013 DRE seemed to have been abandoned, its agenda eroded.

The Care Quality Commission was set up in 2009: part of its remit was to monitor interests of people who had been restricted under the Mental Health Act. They found cultural differences. Among black people, there were a higher proportion of people detained under the Mental Health Act: *"People from all Black and minority ethnic (BME) groups can be overrepresented within inpatient mental health services, and higher rates of people from BME groups are subject to the Act[105].*

Furthermore, at that time, black people appeared to have less access to evidenced-based interventions; black men had more coercive routes into the mental health system. There was variation across communities: figures showed people having their liberty taken away from them and treated against their will. The Count me In Census showed admission rates for black people were six times higher in 2010. Rates for hospitalisation were lower than average for the White British group, but *"were higher than average for all other ethnic groups; they were particularly high for the Black African, Black Caribbean and Other Black groups, who had rates up to two times higher than average."*[106]

The Equality Act was set up in 2010 to promote anti-discrimination. If health care or social care organisations provided goods, facilities or services to the public, they had to ensure they did what the equality law required. This was government legislation on gender, race, disability, sexual orientation, ageing, religion and belief. At the same time service users (people who used the mental health service) spoke out. One said: *"There is disquiet amongst our BAME community about how we are treated by the mental health system; it oppresses us instead of helping us. Instead of helping, it demonizes us, causing us to have to fight for justice all the time. We do not want to be viewed/ treated as victims, but with dignity and respect."*

The government set up a new Mental Health Strategy: '*No Health Without Mental Health*' was launched in February 2011. However, it seemed in the Department of Health, of those responsible for drawing up the Strategy, few came from ethnic minority groups. Not that it should matter, but with poor advisors, the unpalatable discriminatory aspects of mental health, ethnicity and culture seemed to have been erased from the agenda. When questions were raised about the access and treatment of minority groups, the ubiquitous response to any issue under discussion was inevitably '*more research is needed*'.

Data Action Feedback Loop. It appeared that rather than creating a central archive of relevant reports, or acting on appropriate completed research, government ministers wanted 'more research'. This created a cycle of consultation, data collection, report with recommendations, and so on. No one seemed to take responsibility for ensuring evidence based action (like that on which the DRE programme was based). Action was the missing step in the research cycle.

This apparent cycle of 'non intervention' in some parts of Britain suggested we were caught up in patterns of behaviour known as the psychologist Argyris' Ladder of Inference[107]. In this way we became blind to the need to take action based on evidence: we went through a research and consultation process, got caught in a feedback loop, and did not make a decision to manifest action. Perhaps this ensured the main role of government organisations was to maintain status quo?

The ladder illustrated the thinking process we went through, to get from a fact to an action. We tended to observe facts, interpret data according to our beliefs, apply our existing assumptions, develop judgment, then commission more research according to the boundaries of our own knowledge. Yes, I was a biased researcher: all that effort and so little social change. On the positive side, the ladder can be used to help people understand ways they might think differently about an issue. Many organisations do take account of research results, to create social change.

Race Equality is 'Out Of Fashion'

During 2011 a wide gulf appeared between what happened on the ground with mental health and BAME service users, and within government policy. There seemed to be less concern in government circles about racism, accompanied by an assumption that racism was last year's problem. On the one hand, 21st century Britain had a good record with regard to race relations, but appeared to be stuck in a rut regarding mental health issues (although this was hotly denied within certain medical hierarchies). Members of RAWOrg (Rights and Wellbeing of Racialised Groups[108]) pointed out that racism was more prevalent in UK mental health services and Islamophobia in particular. In 2010 the Single Equalities Act covered many areas, of which race and faith were included. However, the political assumption seemed to be that race was 'yesterday's fight'. Ethnicity and health were 'out of fashion'.

In 2011, the Care Quality Commission monitored BAME use of mental health services, but did not appear to have a remit to regulate quality. Representatives from the Afiya Trust (set up to reduce inequalities in health and social care) asked whether the Care Quality Commission could observe the point of service delivery, where there was discrimination for service users. But at that time, discrimination was seen as a local community issue, rather than an institutional problem.

Concerns about mental health, discrimination, and ethnicity were expressed by various organisations. Marcel Vige, chair of RAWOrg commented: *"This issue is not just for NHS providers and commissioning bodies. We need to ensure they commission services in an appropriate way to ensure needs are met. There is a major hurdle with commissioning groups, who do not think race equality is important. The challenges are difficult because equalities and race are not explicit in the government's mental health policy. If we want to have an impact, we need to push it upstream with multi agency working."*

Although sometimes excellent material on cultural beliefs and strategies for addressing mental health were presented, in other organisations ethnicity seemed to be off the agenda, regarding participants and content. For example I attended an all day conference in London, about good practice for mental health recovery. Speakers were excellent, informing about innovative strategies for addressing recovery. I was concerned: I feared certain BAME groups (of new migrants and refugees) would not access services through NHS Foundation Trusts, and neither hear about nor access recovery projects. This aspect of equalities was not touched on.

Then there were those who claimed there was institutional racism within mental health care[109] however, others who worked in the field said it was not helpful to mention it[110]. One who worked with *'an independent Network open to all Black and Minority Ethnic (BAME) people'*[111], said *"the Count Me In census 2010 clearly states that at least for three of the twelve DRE goals nothing has changed and hence there is still an over-representation of BAME people in mental health institutions."*

The arena of cultural competency was complex. Some people claimed race and ethnicity were not an issue in mental health care, while others claimed institutional racism was prevalent. Others seemed to practice 'reverse racism'. Yet other groups claimed there were universal systemic problems of access and aftercare, which existed regardless of one's race or ethnicity. How might we address these conflicting concerns? Myself, I had other unfashionable concerns...

All White, All Right?

Earlier I mentioned a concern about those who drew up and advised on the new government's mental health strategy, were not originally from a variety of different ethnic groups. It is not that I believe a person's ethnicity invariably influences their belief systems and sensitivities, but my concern regarding this deepened during a meeting on the Government's Mental Health Strategy in 2011 where the topic of ethnicity was absent. Although speakers noted the importance of 'an equalities focused approach', they did not expand on what they meant by equalities. During the first 100 minutes of the meeting, I heard no mention of issues around mental health, race and ethnicity.

This meeting about the government strategy for the management of mental health in UK was held at Carlton House Terrace. As it was held under the Chatham House Rule[112], no one participating could be identified. I noticed the word 'disease' was used several times when referring to mental health, a bio-medical term which would not be acceptable to all BAME groups.

Speakers noted stigma was attached to both mental health service users and service providers. Mental health was the largest single cause of disability in UK, costing £105 billion a year, 23% of the total budget. We were told a third of those who consulted general practitioners had illnesses which were mental health related: 25% of those with mental health problems were treated, whereas 90% of patients with physical symptoms were treated.

At the meeting there appeared to be an overwhelming assumption amongst speakers that only one model of mental health was considered by the Department of Health. This was a bio-medical model, with its disease pathology, contained by pharmaceuticals and talking therapies. However, based on UK research evidence, there was a plurality of cultural explanatory models for symptoms of mental distress. If we did not have the humility to acknowledge all citizen's and resident's theories of illness causation, how could we engage equitably with sufferers, meet their perceived needs, and offer inclusion within UK health services? At that evening meeting there was no mention of appropriate interventions which could be used with new migrants and refugees, unfamiliar with pathways to access health care.

During a break one government advisor pronounced that he and his colleagues only read peer reviewed publications to inform the Mental Health Strategy. He did not consider grey literature a resource. This disturbed me. Unpublished (grey) literature included: reports by the Kings Fund; local Primary Care Trusts; research by university and medical school students; charities and advocacy services, many of whom worked on cutting edge projects, with local communities, at the front line.

The government advisor's unwillingness to use unpublished literature meant he ignored a huge resource: evaluation reports in charities and small organisations, written to explain how funding had been used in the community, and its effectiveness, were not used as a source of reference, nor considered appropriate to impact government mental health strategy.

In the last few years, intensive programmes had been conducted by the former Primary Care Trusts concerned about Public Health Issues within their local communities. Reports on evidence based projects on equality and cultural diversity were available, but not consulted. I wondered how many health promotion projects there were across UK, which had undertaken consultation, analysed data, written reports, but which had not been published in peer review journals, and then had their recommendations ignored? There appeared to be no central government archive.

Unmentionable ethnicity. At the Carlton House Terrace meeting, there was no mention of appropriate therapeutic strategies which might be used by people of diverse backgrounds. Based on consultation, I was aware UK residents and citizens from certain cultural backgrounds preferred a group counselling model rather than a western model of 1:1 talking. As in India, they also preferred to use religious or spiritual strategies to address suffering at the same time. At question time I asked about mental health and ethnicity: one speaker responded by saying the Institute of Psychiatry had an anthropologist on their staff, so they were aware of cultural issues. This did not mean that awareness stretched to government offices.

Above all, I was shocked by the unmentionable ethnicity of those attending this meeting in central London. We appeared to be All White. I didn't see any Black or Asian attendees, either as GPs, psychiatrists, members of Department of Health, service users, carers, or politicians. I didn't see anyone of dual or mixed heritage. Was I mistaken? Were we as a group of 100 participants, discussing the government's Mental Health Strategy, representative of the UK population?

I was angry about the ethnic makeup of participants at such an important meeting on Mental Health, with no race equality or diversity on the agenda. The lack of ethnic minorities in attendance disturbed me profoundly: how could such an important event on the Mental Health Strategy occur without input from professionals or experts in the field of mental health, who had an interest in race and culture, equality and diversity? There appeared to be a gap in our understanding of cultural diversity, however, during 2014 the topic of religion, spirituality and mental health returned to the disussion table.

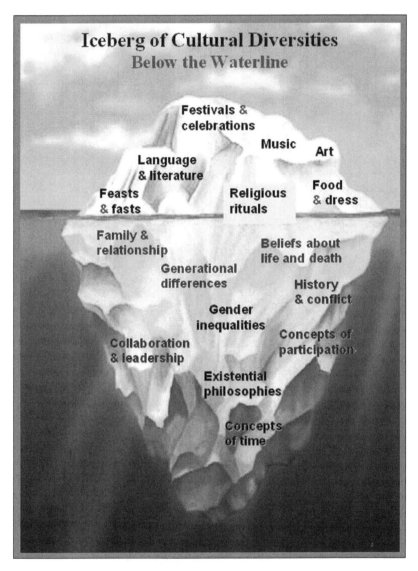

Iceberg of Cultural Diversities

Iceberg Model of Diversity. In UK popular understanding of the term diversity appeared to be just be the tip of an iceberg with other aspects of culture lying below the surface. For example, we had a good understanding of cultural food and dress, feasts and fasts, language and literature, and festivals and celebrations. I wondered to what extent all medical and health care practitioners understood social, cultural and religious factors that determined the health and well-being of their patients. Although we were familiar with superficial popular aspects of culture, we had a poorer understanding of religious rituals, cultural beliefs about life and death, generational differences, family relationships, gender inequalities, and people's history of conflicts and trauma.

Different communities may have quite different existential philosophies about the meaning of life. These philosophies may be hidden, but can be influential regarding people's access to and acceptance of health care treatment. Once we understand deeper aspects of culture in UK, we can better support clients who hold spiritual models of health. More profound understanding would support therapeutic interaction and communication, and result in enhanced social well-being.

Quality of Patient Experience: on the Shelf?

A few months later I attended a meeting on quality run by NHS London and King's Fund, who had developed benchmarking for best practice with mental health care. However, at the meeting it became obvious that the underlying assumption was the only data they needed to collect regarded clinical matters.

Service providers' assumed their services began and ended with clinical intervention. Their benchmarking was about 'captive people' who were already inpatients or outpatients. This was in stark contrast to problems identified by carers and service users, which were about support (or lack of it) <u>before</u> they accessed clinical services, and <u>after</u> they were discharged. The underlying assumption at this meeting on quality, was that social, housing, environmental, or financial issues were of negligible importance to UK mental health. They were not included in the benchmarking model.

During the meeting BAME mental health promotion was not mentioned, nor the need to target religious and community groups, nor any awareness of cultural beliefs influencing access to health care. The main focus of the event was the research, audit, and monitoring of clinical activity.

That was fine, but was it joined up thinking? Was it related to social needs? The quality of patient experience <u>before</u> receiving clinical activity were related to problems of access, and the quality of patient experience <u>after</u> clinical activity were related to continuity of care. The problem was, after treatment, patients returned to the same environment, which triggered distress, and they became revolving door patients. There appeared to be no seamless, co-ordinated, collaborative care.

Research reports which collected data after consultation, seemed to be an end product on a dusty shelf, rather than evidence based material on which to negotiate appropriate social or medical change. The feedback loop appeared to stop: data collection, followed by report recommendations, followed by inaction. This was not always the case, but it was demoralising when it happened.

In 2013 NHS London was renamed the London Strategic Health Authority for the London Region. On 1st April 2013 the Clinical Commissioning Groups came into being, made up of local GPs and health professionals. In Harrow some of their offices can be found at the site of the former NHS Harrow: some Primary Care Trust staff were redeployed, so their expertise in public health was not entirely lost.

That year, during a CCG Harrow Public Drop-in Event a GP speaker said their one aim was to reduce inequalities (unspecified), and one of their principles was seamless patient care. The NHS was now monitored by the Care Quality Commission and the consumer champion Healthwatch Harrow. There seemed to be an embarrassment around the topic of racial inequalities, even to talk about it in a borough like Harrow, in which the census showed ethnic minority groups were in the majority. Mentioning race and ethnicity felt taboo.

Currently there are newly named practitioners (AMHP[113]) involved in decisions about mental health disorders and compulsory detention in England and Wales: these practitioners may be community psychiatric nurses, social workers, occupational therapists, and psychologists. By 2013, the former Delivering Race Equality agenda seemed to have been forgotten, and the new mental health strategy covered a wider range of equalities, among which was included race equality.

However, in spite of the government equalities agenda, detention for Black and Minority Ethnic groups under the Mental Health Act had not declined and these groups were still over represented within psychiatric institutions[114]. Many groups in UK were asking for race equality to be put back on the agenda for mental health. During 2014 religion and health started to come back on the agenda.

However, denial and cultural blindness about ethnicity and mental health were not the only issues to concern me: there were also problems with different frameworks of understanding about health, and different ways of interpreting symptoms of distress. People had different models and cultural worldviews about reality. I tackle these issues in the next section.

Section Two Eurocentrism and Paradigm Problems

A paradigm is a model or worldview. In addition to state government denial about problems with culture, ethnicity and mental health, I noted other concerns which came from paradigm problems:

- Eurocentric and indigenous frameworks of understanding health
- Different cultural interpretations of distress
- Culture bound models: Western and Asian

However, there was an awareness of paradigm problems at local government levels, by some mental health professionals, and in some academic environments. This was not universally the case with all front line service providers.

Models: Eurocentric and Indigenous

There are additional complexities involved when addressing the topic of mental health. Different cultural frameworks of understanding the world and human existence are not always compatible. Eurocentric and indigenous models of health may be at odds with each other. In UK medical and health care practitioners, patients and their carers may hold quite different ways of understanding reality. One person's objective knowledge may be focused around 'ordinary waking consciousness' and post natal experiences, while another's knowledge may focus on direct cognition and pre-natal experiences.

In addition, throughout the world, cultural interpretations of symptoms of distress are variable. Our understanding of the terms 'normal' and 'deviant' are culturally sensitive, and even within western culture, concepts of them change throughout history. The phrase 'common consensus' also changes over time, and is usually dependant on the beliefs of one's peers or a ruling elite. The diagnosis, treatment and healing modalities presented in this book illustrate a wide range of what is considered 'normal'.

Since its origins, the main aim of psychiatry was to reduce individual human suffering. In the western world, psychiatry (a 19th century term) was a medical practice concerned with diagnosing, treating and preventing mental, emotional, and behavioural conditions. In India psychiatrists and psychologists were educated in western models of diagnosis and treatment, and were examined by western exam boards. However there was increasing frustration amongst some Indian professionals, when they observed local syncretic practices and treatment strategies, which they perceived to be effective at addressing human suffering[115]. These spiritual psychiatries were rarely formally taught or examined in India, although in UK there are exceptions[116].

The preceding chapters presented a series of frameworks and models of understanding about body, health, and universe, which are quite different from a western biomedical model of health. The consultation rituals and types of collaboration between medical and religious practitioners and indigenous healers were presented, together with syncretic and plural health seeking strategies for mental distress. We might assume multiple health seeking strategies do not occur in the west, but research in London illustrated otherwise[117]. The chapters set out cultural explanatory models and theories of illness causation, and the ways these influenced people's interpretation of their symptoms. In UK these cultural models also co-existed with bio-medical explanations of illness.

This book presented treatment strategies which were generated as a result of diagnosis according to a particular theory of causation. It also discussed explanations of treatments, by presenting informants' descriptions of their healing mechanisms and modalities. The manuscript emphasised the importance of beliefs: the ways they influenced our understanding of the human 'self' both as an individual and within society. It discussed various specialists' philosophies of existence, health and medicine, and their knowledge about the nature of reality and consciousness.

Paradigm problems may occur when there are dominant models of health, diagnosis and treatment, alongside key cultural differences regarding beliefs on the nature of human existence. This occurred particularly when the dominant model of medicine and health care was biological, and front line staff did not make room for spiritual models. Although religion and faith were frequently acknowledged, these concerned rituals or calendars: discrete beliefs about human existence and health that co-existed at the same time were rarely mentioned. There is still room in UK front line practice for additional insights and cultural humility.

One key problem in developing transferable models from data gathered in India, to populations residing within Britain, is the need to acknowledge and understand different paradigms of health, different types of knowledge[118], and the role of cultural humility.

In UK, there tended to be one dominant model of health and medicine: a biological interpretation of symptoms, and subsequent treatment strategies that usually involved pharmacological solutions, with a possibility of talking therapy. In India a plurality of health seeking strategies coexisted contemporaneously. The population's interpretation of their symptoms, and the meanings they gave, both influenced the diagnosis they would accept, and the treatment they were offered.

In India professionals seemed to hold multiple models of body and health at the same time. They accepted their patients used different practitioners for their treatment, and indeed referred them to religious and spiritual practitioners.

Research indicated some ethnic groups in UK were underserved by the health care authorities[119]. Their cultural differences influenced their access to services[120]. It would make a significant difference if healthcare providers had a deeper understanding of cultural expressions of physical and mental distress. For example in UK, there were many cultural explanatory models for triggers of mental illness, and these are set out in the chart below. They included biomedical and psychological triggers; environmental triggers and social conflict; substance abuse; being at the effect of someone else's inappropriate behaviour. There were many supernatural theories of illness causation, and these included: unusual experiences and visions; spirit possession and ghosts; effects of Karma, ancestral misbehaviour, past lives, and reincarnation. There were also planetary influences at the time of birth, or at the time of illness; experiences of religious malpractice; effect of non-local consciousness and subtle energy on mental wll-being.

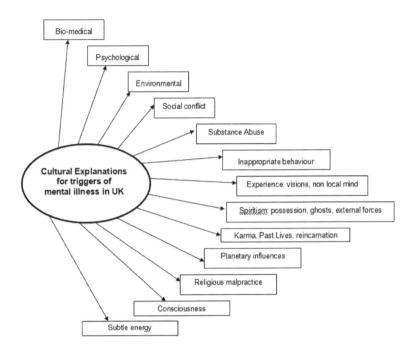

Cultural Explanations of Triggers

Understanding BAME Perspectives in UK

How do we grasp BAME perspectives in mental health, when the topic seems taboo, and when culture bound blindness seems to exist among Department of Health hierarchies? The philosophies recorded in India are transferable to the communities in towns and cities in UK with populations of diverse ethnicity. The data illustrates that the underlying assumption of only one model of health, is disproved by the plural models and philosophies UK populations hold[121], [122].

The London Borough of Harrow, where I conducted research, has one of the most ethnically diverse populations in UK.

There are now NHS initiatives which take religious and spiritual practices into consideration[123], [124], and although innovations are taking place in some areas, extended use of cultural frameworks to understand mental distress would benefit more UK patients. BAME groups are questioning current psychiatric and mental health care practices in UK, and people are emphasising the relevance of ethnicity issues and want government policy makers to address it, in particular regarding deeper cultural awareness of front line mental health practitioners.

One problem seemed to be: there was significant awareness of cultural frameworks of health among those who studied trans-cultural psychiatry or medical anthropology. There was a wide range of scholarly literature on library bookshelves, about cultural philosophies and cultural models of health.

The problem was that this knowledge did not filter into the educational curricula of many front line health and social care providers.

In UK it seemed as if we maintained two parallel types of expertise: the clinical medical model and cultural models. One was taught to front line staff, the other taught to academics and scholars. In my opinion, this division was inappropriate.

There was a need for the topic to be addressed immediately within educational medical and health care core curricula, and as part of post registration training. However, according to Gail Hornstein the problem in mental health went deeper than cultural misunderstandings.

Frameworks of Understanding.

On the dust jacket of her book, Gail Hornstein[125] wrote: *"A vast gulf exists between the way medicine explains psychiatric illness and the experiences of those who suffer."* The gulf she spoke about was not one relating to understanding BAME knowledge frameworks, but the gulf between medical interpretations of illness and disease versus 'service user' or 'survivor' interpretation of triggers of symptoms.

When she spoke to mental health patients, their narratives were not only about their experiences, but they were proposing different ways of understanding their symptoms. They wanted to escape their doctor's narrow thinking, reframe psychological issues, and engage in the possibility of recovery. She found some were weaning themselves off medication, and attending peer support groups, rather than day centres.

Hornstein stressed the important role of life experiences in causing depression, and questioned claims about 'chemical imbalance', as being 'only one point of view'. Like Moncrieff[126], Watters[127], and Stastny[128] she wondered why society had medicalised mental health to such an extent. The narratives of former in-patients in British psychiatric institutions echo these views[129].

Whose Culture Bound Models?

In India there was a wide range of cultural explanations for triggers of mental distress, beliefs which were also held by Asian populations in UK. These explanatory models were set out in the figure on preceding page. It was important to acknowledge the many different explanatory models because a person's theories of illness causation influenced their health seeking strategies, and their acceptance of diagnoses and treatment.

We understand from previous chapters that people's theories of illness causation were generated within different paradigms, and healing modalities, sometimes contemporaneously.

In some cases, when professionals heard about explanations which did not fit their own belief system, they may have thought they were culture bound. Alternatively, they may have accepted different theories of illness causation, because they understood peoples' beliefs influenced their access to a wide range of healthcare diagnosis and treatment.

Practitioners may not have understood some explanations such as arguments about non-local mind, or pre-natal experiences, or may have suggested they were wrong or delusional. Other beliefs included survival beyond death, the role of karma, astrology, or spiritism, which practitioners may also have felt were culture bound, while retaining their own existential culture bound belief systems. Or, these beliefs may already be part of practitioner's existential realities, which they hold alongside their acceptance of clinical practices.

In the following section, I present projects for mental well being, which were set up in the London Borough of Harrow, in order to explore in greater detail the relevance of data collected in India for UK populations.

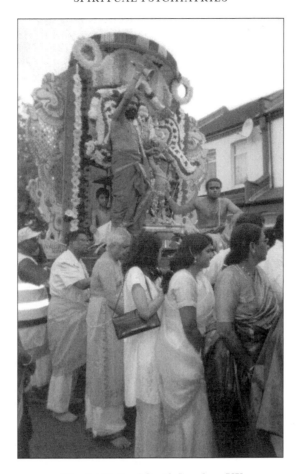

Chariot Festival South London, UK

Section Three: London Borough of Harrow

The London borough of Harrow has one of the most ethnically diverse populations in UK. Of its residents, 69% belong to diverse ethnic groups, and 30% are Asian or Asian British. Given the ethnicity of the population, the borough health services used particular strategies to address the mental health needs of those who were migrants and refugees. I will explore the extent to which Indian treatment strategies presented in earlier chapters, might be transferable to a UK context.

According to census figures, over one third of Harrow's residents were born abroad, coming from 203 different countries, including Iran, Afghanistan, Eastern Europe, Somalia, and Middle East. Those born outside UK have different needs from those of the same ethnicity born within the UK. This means healthcare professionals need to consider ways of working with different ethnic groups, and different generations of those ethnic groups. When patients present for a consultation, first, second and third generations may look ethnically the same, may practice the same religion, and wear the same clothing style, but may be quite different culturally and morally.

During 2009 and 2010, a series of projects under the title of Bridging Cultures and Dissolving Barriers[130] were commissioned by NHS Harrow with a local mental health charity. The remit was to explore mental health promotion with black and minority ethnic groups. During a needs assessment exercise, religious and community leaders had emphasised the importance of religion and faith for their mental well-being. The aim of the project was two-fold: to address health inequalities and inequalities of access to mental health services for service users, and to raise awareness about cultural and religious understanding of mental health with service providers.

As part of the project I ran seminar events using a participatory approach, working with community and faith leaders to deliver outcomes. Medical and allied health and social care professionals were encouraged to participate in the delivery of seminars. The result meant participants gained improved self-management of their mental health and had better access to services through their increased understanding of Western diagnostic terms. In this way it was hoped that an early deterioration of mental health was prevented. Healthcare providers became more aware of minority concerns about mental health in particular.

During that project I became aware people forced into migration from their country of origin, or from places where their ancestors were buried, may be more at risk of experiencing episodes of stress, anxiety or mental ill health. Forced migration was the result of war or trauma, or holding beliefs which were incompatible with a country's ruling parties, and had resulted in imprisonment. Living away from the support of extended family and friends could also increase social isolation. Religious and spiritual practices were of great importance especially for first generation migrants.

As a project facilitator I felt it important to acknowledge people's beliefs about illness causation as this influenced their health seeking strategies, and their access to services. Their beliefs about stigma and mental health influenced what they did to get help. It was obvious people's beliefs about existence influenced how they explained the symptoms of mental distress and their seeking access to care. Beliefs about the meaning of symptoms were quite different in different cultures, and some symptoms were interpreted as requiring treatment from religious practitioners, rather than from clinical practitioners. Hindu people preferred to ask priests to chant the ancient Sanskrit Mrityunjay Mantra, to awaken healing forces in body, mind, and soul.

During seminar discussions with Asian populations in Harrow, it became clear that religious and spiritual practices were important aspects of daily life: they supported social cohesion and cultural memories, and helped people find meaning in their life. When people felt anxious or upset they tended to visit religious organisations alongside healthcare professionals. Furthermore there was a problem of stigma relating to mental health, as symptoms of distress could be seen as a sign of weakness. This meant people tended to remain silent about it or developed psychosomatic physical symptoms instead of emotional ones. For some BAME people the concept of mental health itself was alien, as people had different beliefs about the body and the self.

Religious and Community Leaders in Harrow explained that creating understanding about mental health was a two-way process. To address this two way process, events were run: to increase cultural understanding among staff, and to support access to mental healthcare services among BAME groups.

Challenging Stigma in Harrow

Time to Change project was launched in 2009, to challenge mental health stigma and discrimination, and overturn generations of prejudice. Their vision was to end mental health discrimination, and they developed a powerful media campaign to change attitudes. Time to Change representatives said 90% of mental health patients still reported discrimination. In 2011, they focused a campaign on Asian people in Harrow.

Six key findings[131] of Time to Change research were:
- Shame, fear and secrecy surround mental illness
- The causes of mental illness are often misunderstood
- The family can be both caring and isolating
- Social pressure to conform
- People with mental health problems are not valued
- Marriage prospects can be damaged by mental illness

Their objectives were to: improve knowledge, attitudes and behaviour towards people with mental health problems within the South Asian community in Harrow; and use measurable results to learn more about what works to change knowledge, attitudes and behaviour within this specific BAME population. Time to Change focused their admirable project on reducing stigma and discrimination towards mental health amongst Asian populations. However, in my opinion, this was just one strand of the problem: there was still an outstanding need to develop deeper cultural awareness among staff.

Care Programme Approach, Harrow

The social marketing campaign by Time to Change did go some way to addressing stigma with the South Asian community, but there were still problems between service users and carers and service providers. There were cultural issues to consider, and universal concerns regarding access to mental health care and support.

Appendix B illustrates one example of the way in which a package of strategies developed on paper in an NHS health care trust office was ideal, but did not meet the actual needs of patients on the ground in practice. The Care Programme set out how a mental health patient's package of NHS and social support worked collaboratively together. However, in practice, there appeared to be differences between the experiences of Asian service users and carers in Harrow, and those in NHS offices who developed services.

I attended an EKTA meeting for South Asian people, run by Chandra Shah. Details in Appendix B illustrate differences of understanding between a representative of a local NHS Trust, and actual Asian mental health patients. I have included it because these differences did not relate to cultural differences of belief or interpretation, or paradigm differences, nor cultural world views, but simply to access of mental health services.

Also in Harrow, Rethink Support Group was an organisation that helped people affected by severe mental illness recover a better quality of life. Carers attending Rethink meetings expressed deep anger at the Care Programme Approach. One person claimed the CPA was just a piece of paper without value: they claimed staff were monitored as to whether or not they had filled it out, but there was no evidence or audit of any action taken. I realised that access to Care Programme Assessment services was not merely an Asian or BAME cultural issue. It was a universal mental health service user and carer issue.

Participants at Rethink wanted a complete change of belief, to one that recovery from mental ill health was possible. This has now changed, due to the work of two pioneers: Margaret McHugh and Gary Butcher, who developed the Confidence for Life programme, and inspired by them the NHS Trust in question (CNWL[132]) established its own 'Recovery Colleges'.

Whilst writing this chapter, I attended a meeting of Rethink Harrow, to celebrate their 30 year anniversary. Carers were still angry about the treatment of their relatives within the mental health care system. They were concerned newly formed GP commissioners would make wrong decisions if they followed the Department of Health's mental health care strategy. The

Commissioners were responsible for medical policy, and the Local Authority for social care. On the surface this was appropriate, but it didn't work in practice for service users, some of whom claimed they did not have care co-ordinators. Although issues around mental health care were clearly not only a BAME problem, Black and Asian Minority Ethnic group service users and carers experienced particular problems.

Culture Bound Denial

The mental health service problems experienced by Black and Asian Ethnic Minority groups were highlighted in an internet discussion which took place during 2013. A report had been published[133] in June, which created much critical comment, and it was claimed the government had managed to control both the data and the results. Some respondents said the data fitted well within current political frameworks, others denounced it as flawed research.

The report in question produced evidence to suggest ethnicity had nothing to do with being sectioned under the Mental Health Act 1983. This set up a fast and furious debate among scholars, NHS staff, and psychiatrists on the Minority Ethnic Health email list.[134] Members acknowledged, since the end of the Delivering Race Equality programme, ethnic inequalities in mental health services were not a Department of Health priority.

However, evidence was submitted to this email group, that not only were people from black ethnic groups at higher risk of detention, but also *"black patients are perceived to be more dangerous despite lower ratings of psychopathology.*[135]*"* The psychiatrist Suman Fernando commented: *"The wider issues are that black people are still suffering in the psychiatric services, especially at the hard end and there is a need to develop if possible a public debate"*. A suggestion was made to set up a more profound review of ethnicity and compulsory detention, and to liaise with All-Party Parliamentary Groups for both Race and Community, and Mental Health on the topic of ethnic inequalities.

Why was there a mismatch between the general population, and the ethnicity of those detained under section? Some carers suggested there was misdiagnosis of their relatives, together with institutional racism. Others suggested there were different ways of manifesting symptoms (e.g. psychosomatic), and different ways of interpreting those symptoms (spiritual). They were agreed about the damaging effects of stigma and discrimination, both within family and community, and within the healthcare system itself.

Although issues around cultural competency were clearly known about at an academic level: at the level of front line practitioners, awareness seemed to be rather ad hoc. Cultural humility to find out about a patient's beliefs was not universally practiced. That quite simply was not good enough. Later some London boroughs began to run training in cultural humility and communication for front line staff.

Section Four Communication: a Reflexive Approach

In the previous section I suggested it was not essential for service providers to hold the same belief system as their clients, although it was helpful to suspend judgement, work together and communicate beliefs from each person's perspective, and then arrive at a negotiated treatment strategy. The data suggest the importance of cultural humility and negotiated communication in a therapeutic environment.

In the 1980s Kleinman, an American psychiatrist and medical anthropologist had suggested systematic ways of enquiring about a patient's explanatory models[136], so practitioner and client could reach a negotiated solution about treatment. However, over 30 years later, this is still not universally taught as part of the curriculum in UK, although it is taught in American medical schools.

In UK, psychiatrists Bhui and Bhugra explored explanatory models for mental ill health and their implications for clinical practice[137]. They suggested patients were more satisfied if practitioners understood their models of health and wrote:

"It may be that the explanatory paradigm of psychiatrists, which has a predominantly biomedical orientation, explains the hesitation with which social science methods are absorbed into routine psychiatric practice. The 'process' of enquiry is crucial to social scientists and should be of prime important in clinical psychiatric practice. Yet rarely does clinical practice systematically apply the process rules to elicit explanatory models and to maximise collaboration and communication between patient and professional".

In the past some medical practitioners believed illness could be cured by treating symptoms with pharmacology alone, without addressing a patient's belief about illness causation[138]. The problem: when clinical diagnosis and treatment are given a high value, this may result in the meaning of the illness to the patient being ignored.

Psychiatrists Bhui and Bhugra suggested practitioners learn about earlier stages of a person's experience of illness and their cultural explanatory models for distress. It would be excellent if more teaching colleges would address the gap in UK between knowledge obtained from academic research, and its practical application for frontline medical, social, and health care staff. Bhui's transcultural psychiatry courses at Wolfson Institute, at Queen Mary's in London, set an encouraging example, as did Littlewood's course at University College London. This was important training about transcultural psychiatry, as were recommendations in a position statement by the Royal College of Psychiatrists[139], but these needed to be offered and taken up more widely by front line practitioners.

Communication and Quality.

Communication was an important factor to get right, both at an individual level, and at a societal level. It may sound simple, but care needed to be taken to ensure communication between practitioners and patients was mutually understandable. Medical and healthcare workers needed to collaborate to enhance sharing of information. Although I was aware there were policies to address this, I was unsure to what extent the practice of collaboration was audited, to ensure effectiveness, for service users, carers, and service providers. Concordance of understanding of belief system between practitioner and patient improved potential for healing. This was the same in UK or in India.

In India the ancient medical herbalists took a holistic view of mental health. In UK, cases where mental ill health was triggered by external circumstances, practitioners still needed to ensure there was an effective continuity of communication and collaboration between social workers, housing, medical, and health care providers. It sounded obvious: in principle the strategies already existed and were in place.

Seamless collaborative health care was part of the new CCG's vision (Clinical Commissioning Group), but what did it mean in practice? When a person experienced mental distress, it may be their circumstances which needed to be addressed in a practical manner, alongside pharmacology. In theory this should have been dealt with as part of a person's care plan, but in practice it was clear from meetings I later attended, that this was not always the case.

These considerations of communication, humility and collaboration were essential for medical and health care practitioners who worked in multicultural societies, to gain deeper understanding of their patients' beliefs about the causes of mental illness.

Cultural Diversity Upstream.

Seamless upstream healthcare for social benefit was a concept embraced by GP Dr Chris Manning. His suggested approach was to travel *"upstream as far as possible to help people to deal with the causes of their problems and predicaments, rather than simply seeing them as patients with diagnoses and becoming tied up in medical corsetry. Going Upstream means being tough on the causes of problems and predicaments and not just working on down- stream consequences"[140]*.

I wondered how far upstream we needed to go, to create policies of fundamental change within mental health care education in the UK. Upstream thinking considered the social, economic, and environmental origins of health: it looked for root causes of ill health and real solutions.

Upstream healthcare was key to enhance the well being of the nation: this meant addressing and acknowledging the evidence based triggers of distress and disturbance, rather than simply clinically treating the symptoms, then sending a person back to the same environment. However, this required a change of paradigm thinking: and a willingness to acknowledge that external factors played a fundamental role in mental heath and well being.

Chapter Fourteen

TRANSFERABLE STRATEGIES IN PRACTICE

In this book I presented data from interviews with mental health practitioners in India, and from meetings about mental health which I attended in London, UK. I wanted to explore what principles there were in common, and what learning might be possible by discussing mental health practices in each country.

In India I used a snowballing ethnographic research strategy. Serendipity met scholarship and played a significant role in where I went and who I interviewed. I am aware the doctors and psychiatrists I met at Pondicherry were particularly if not extremely sensitive to spiritual matters. They held explicit views about spirituality and psychiatric or psychological practices. These views influenced their practice and their teaching. In spite of this bias, I wanted to know whether an ideal set of principles might be proposed, and whether there were transferable strategies that might be used to manifest effective therapeutic healing benefit to UK populations.

I have set out various themes below, and made suggestions as to what might be suitable to consider with western populations, whatever their ethnicity. I noted earlier in the chapter, that there were some considerations in UK specific to Black and Asian populations, whereas strategies used by certain local authority mental health programmes appeared universally problematic regardless of ethnicity.

In the UK the current government had a vision for seamless collaborative mental healthcare, but this was not necessarily what happened in practice, according to academic observers, practitioners, service users and carers. Effective multi-agency care was the ideal, but not always the actual practice. The final comments below suggest ways to enhance the mental healthcare experience of patients, carers, and practitioners themselves. The underlying assumption is that a spiritual approach to mental health care is desirable and feasible.

Consultation, Collaboration and Communication

The normal practice I observed in India was for consultation with a psychiatrist to involve the individual person with mental distress, plus their family members, carers, and student social workers. Furthermore it was normal practice for collaboration to occur between medical, religious and alternative practitioners. In UK the normal practice for consultation with a psychiatrist involved the individual with mental distress, plus perhaps a translator or advocate, although in Care Plan meetings there may be many more professionals present. With patient consent, BAME (Black and Asian Minority Ethnic) family members would like to be present at a consultation. Recent research indicated in some cases group counselling was preferred, rather than one to one.

It is appropriate for organisations to consider culturally appropriate consultation and counselling. Elsewhere in the world, the controlled public acknowledgement of distress and disturbance has been found to be healing[141]. With negotiation, it would be possible to check with UK clients, to discuss whether they prefer one-to-one individual meetings, or one including family and advisors.

Collaboration. In India, it was normal for people to consult different practitioners: they engaged in contemporaneous or sequential consultation and shared advice. Patients collaborated with biomedical, psychological, complimentary, religious and spiritual practitioners. Although people took pharmaceutical drugs for their mental distress, they also visited other practitioners who performed religious or 'traditional' rituals. Patients and their relatives considered there was a benefit to plural health seeking strategies, as each therapy targeted different aspects of an illness.

In UK Care Plan meetings were attended by different kinds of staff, these might include: ward manager, social worker, or housing officer. In the past, a chaplain or religious leader was rarely present. Given the importance of religion and faith to many BAME people, it may be productive for a patient's well being, with consent, to systematically include faith workers. Certain London NHS Trusts like CNWL are already training chaplains in mental health. As well as effective multi-agency working, patients may benefit from collaboration with other practitioners, who offer complementary or spiritual treatments.

Communication Strategies. In UK service providers and their clients do not need to hold the same belief systems, but it may help communication and benefit healing to acknowledge and discuss each person's model of belief, and arrive at a negotiated treatment strategy. This is increasingly referred to as 'cultural humility', rather than cultural competency. Training in effective and reflective communication strategies with the aim of achieving humility would be of social benefit.

❖❖❖

Triggers and Theories of Illness Causation

Throughout the world, peoples' explanatory models for triggers of distress mean they have a variety of ways to interpret their symptoms. There are plural theories of illness causation, and subsequently this results in people choosing many different ways of treating symptoms.

In India practitioners said their patients' triggers for mental distress included problems of relationship, loss, and environment. Staff tended to ask holistic questions about triggers, including historical, spiritual or supernatural theories of illness causation. The doctors interviewed in Pondicherry India claimed physical illness was the last stage of the manifestation of inner disharmony.

In UK we are taught about a range of triggers for illness in general which include physiological, emotional and mental disharmony. Acknowledgement of multiple theories of illness causation, and multiple treatment strategies would help patients contextualise illness in their own personal and cultural terms. Like those NHS Trusts with best practice, we could systematically ask questions to determine what every patient's illness meant to them.

Stigma and Recovery. Some practitioners in Pondicherry assumed mental distress was an episodic event, rather than an illness for life. Recovery was assumed, and in theory this meant there was less stigma attached to a person exhibiting symptoms. Furthermore, physical somatisation of symptoms meant patients experienced less stigma. With regard to the symptoms claimed due to spirit possession in India or UK, it meant those who believed in it considered it was much less a person's responsibility, than if they exhibited symptoms of emotional or mental distress (without apparent cause). It was less stigmatising. In UK, attitudes are shifting and we are now revisiting the proposition that symptoms of mental ill health are episodic, and recovery is possible. The concept of a recovery model was user-led and is increasingly mainstream.

Cultural Therapies and Treatments

Globally in many countries, humans practice a variety of health seeking strategies at the same time: they use plural syncretic treatments to address mental distress. The treatments people select are influenced by their theories of illness causation. This may mean they believe treatments have different healing mechanisms and modalities. For example allopathic medicine or pharmacology may be used at the same time or sequentially as herbal medicine, flower remedies or homoeopathy. Or people may attend religious institutions for prayers, ritual bathing, or commission prophylactic amulets.

There was an assumption that allopathic drugs treated the symptoms of mental distress whereas prayer addressed the causes of those symptoms. Similarly the religious cleric I interviewed suggested Indian psychiatrists treated symptoms, while religious practitioners treated the cause. In UK these and similar beliefs are usually held by first generation migrants in particular.

It would benefit BAME patients in UK if we encouraged prayer and religious rituals where appropriate.[142] Psychiatrists like Dinesh Bughra have acknowledged the importance of patient visits to temple, church and mosque. There are others who accept the role of religious learned men and women in bereavement counselling and performing rituals for the dead.

Evidence gained from the Bridging Cultures project in Harrow UK, suggested it was important for Black and Ethnic Minority groups to benefit from a combination of strategies to address distress, that is, pharmacology, religious ritual, and prayers. It was important to honour personal beliefs, in their influence both on patient health seeking strategies and on staff treatment preferences. It would be useful to generate more research on effectiveness, into which treatments and healing practices work, and whether or to what extent people benefit from the health seeking strategies they use.

Healing Modalities. Western practitioners do already take on board their patients' cultural and religious practices. It would be a small step for staff to acknowledge that different treatments had different healing modalities which might be used at the same time. Research in India indicated it would benefit patients to be offered varying treatments that act at a physical level, mental level, emotional level, and spiritual level. However, I wonder whether the same strategies in UK might require a considerable paradigm shift for some practitioners trained in biomedical therapeutics.

In Pondicherry various psychiatrists I spoke to agreed that different remedies appeared to influence different aspects of a person: pharmacology influenced physical symptoms as did herbal remedies, however homoeopathy in minute doses, invited the body to respond with its own healing, whereas flower remedies directly healed with the soul and spirit of a person. These frameworks of knowledge from Pondicherry doctors are transferable to UK, as doctors belonging to certain organisations[143] would testify. Amongst some GPs there is intellectual space to discuss specific Indian knowledge about the different healing modalities of different treatments, and ways that they work with different parts of the human being. Some UK doctors are already collaborating with practitioners who use treatments with differing healing modalities.

I wonder how far the discussion on healing modalities might comfortably extend. Would it include other therapeutic practices like: prayer, past life therapies, karma, effect of the moon, and reduced medication dosage? Would doctors accept the use of prophylactic amulets as religious or spiritual symbols, simply because some UK patients believed strongly in them? In the following section I explore existential paradigms of the accepted boundaries of knowledge, which influence health practice.

❖ ❖ ❖

Existential Paradigms

Our beliefs about the nature of reality are sometimes so strong, and so deeply embedded, that they are invisible to us. This may mean it is difficult to accept other people's beliefs as knowledge. Existential beliefs may concern our notions of self and identity, or our grasp of the wider faculties of a human being or their experience. The boundaries of knowledge are usually mediated through hierarchy or a dominant world view, as are the concepts of what is normal or abnormal. In Chapter Ten, we saw how colonial, Eurocentric philosophies of existence were maintained in India. Our own culture bound philosophies influence our understanding of health, medicine, spirituality and treatment.

I wondered whether paradigms about the nature of reality, and the nature of human existence were transferable. Different population groups held different beliefs about reality. In the west, the mainstream belief seemed to be that human beings were born, lived one life, then died, and that was the end, unless we went to heaven, hell, or purgatory. There was an underlying Western assumption that we had one life only, and this belief meant within psychiatry some practitioners assumed patients with functional disorders could only be influenced by post natal experiences.

In my opinion, when working with people from BAME groups, it would be more appropriate to use broader strategies for understanding human suffering. Our perspective could be widened to explore patient's views around pre-natal experiences, karma, the planets, evil eye, and curses. It was not that staff needed to agree with these beliefs, but person-centred communication strategies and cultural humility would ensure that if asked, a patient felt heard and understood, and an agreed negotiated treatment solution would become more feasible.

Spirituality questionnaires have already been developed, which could be adapted if necessary and used to explore patient beliefs and religious practices, and their multiple theories of illness causation. It would be beneficial for us to understand the continuum between psychosis and spirituality, healing or negative visionary and auditory experiences, and the changing concept of normality.

The concepts of normal and abnormal are influenced by place, context, by rural and urban situations, by dominant culture, by hierarchies of power, and by geographical location. There is room for further discussion into the nature of the concepts of normal and delusional, which seem to change according to geographical location, time, and personal relationship. These are the subject of a future publication by the author.

Different concepts of self. In India the 'human self' can mean an individual human, the family, the social group, or the extended self as part of a geographical community. In UK, the self tends to mean the individual self, except among members of Black and Asian minority groups, where it can expand to the range of meanings given in India and Africa.

Our sense of self may be changeable, together with our occupational identity, or in relation to our families. In addition, for Indian women with mental health problems, it can mean the family 'self' is shamed or stigmatised. In the following section I consider human existential models, and a range of experiences that human beings claim to have.

Human Experiences and Faculties

Different countries and different societies may have quite different beliefs about existence, consciousness, and the nature of being human. It is an obvious statement. In the same way that our understanding of the human self is culturally determined, so is our understanding of the nature of human faculties like clairvoyance; psychic ability; visual and auditory experiences; communication with spirits; non-local mind, and expanded, and remote perception.

These all require understanding from within a new paradigm. What can humans really do? What experiences can humans actually have? The label we put on experiences depends on our belief system, and the belief system and common consensus of our peers. In general common consensus changes over time and place: what we agree on as 'correct reality' one year, we may change our views a decade later.

There is more than one framework for understanding visionary and auditory experiences. Humans have different levels of perception: it may require quite a shift for some of us to accept the presence of different types of vision, let alone different types of presence. There are those who see mundane reality, those who see subtle beings, and those who see non-local remote events.

A more open understanding of 'normal' events might alter our ways of responding to people who have visionary experiences. It may be that staff are aware of subtle perceptions, and the non-material realities of altered states of consciousness, but may not mention this to colleagues in Western clinical settings.

Training for front line staff would usefully open a discourse on the nature of reality, and the nature of human existence. In a multicultural society like Britain, we have every reason to use education to become familiar with more than one model of reality.

Frameworks of Knowledge

In India the teachers of philosophy I spoke to were intellectually frustrated because they had experienced unequal hierarchies of knowledge. Teachers felt the dominant western model of colonial philosophy prevailed. In UK, apart from transcultural psychiatrists and transpersonal psychologists, medical and health care staff tended to accept the dominance of a Western model of mental health. For example many assumed only post natal experiences could influence mental health. However the Indian model of mental health suggested a variety of different influences including: pre-natal experiences, the role of planets, past lives, karma, spirit possession, negative forces, or positive forces or energy that is either brought down to earth or can be tapped into on earth, similar to some kind of celebrity charisma.

In UK it would be very relevant for practitioners to become familiar with more than one framework of health and body, when working with patients from Black and Asian minority ethnic groups. Or, to develop cultural humility where they could open a discussion to determine a patient is heard, and the treatment offered is meaningful to them.

Furthermore as well as differences in types of 'acceptable' human experiences, there is a fundamental difference between ways of understanding death and the body. Some people assume we die with the body: others say the body is temporary and when it dies our spirit or psychic being continues or survives beyond. Our beliefs about death and survival influence our theories of mental illness causation, and how we treat patients.

Training and Exam Boards

There is a presupposition that in the Western world we manage and control the boundaries of acceptable knowledge. In order to address the educational inequalities in hierarchies of knowledge identified during interviews with the Indian philosophers, exam board requirements would need to be addressed to make allowance for cultural perceptions. In this way students in India and UK can be trained to learn about a range of culturally appropriate psychology and philosophy.

In India, one lecturer of philosophy explained there appeared to be a fundamental difference of understanding, where students of one culture were being examined according to the educational knowledge base of another culture, and the two frameworks of knowledge were not connected.

He explained that his students' learning developed from being examined on western cultural grounds. He said this was totally false: *"when I teach, I feel I'm teaching something very superficial. It has no connexion with the student's soul nor with their individuality. I teach because I need the salary.* "Is it not time for old colonial beliefs about the correctness of knowledge to dissolve, both in India and UK?

Ideal world? New training is needed to acknowledge and raise awareness of the gaps in understanding between mental health patient and practitioner, and to deliver appropriate communication strategies, to enable mutual understanding, and negotiated treatments. Educational seminars would discuss the multiple understandings of the existential nature of the self, and plural understandings of the nature of reality. They could be used to open discussion about the kinds of topics we accept as knowledge of philosophy. Currently it seems only Western cultural knowledge counts as philosophy. Surely there is room for academic hierarchies to accept and examine students in appropriate Indian cultural knowledge? Exam boards need to be revisited to explore whether they are promoting knowledge from colonial or Eurocentric ideologies.

New courses would continue the work of the Royal Collage of Psychiatrists, to introduce the role of spirituality so not only academic psychiatrists were aware but all front-line practitioners; training for practitioners would be offered in multiple theories of illness causation. We would address long standing concerns, and ensure that not only religion, but also race equality and cultural diversity are back on the agenda for mental health care in UK.

These new courses would help to raise awareness of Eurocentric ways of thinking about the causality of ill health. It is particularly relevant in today's multicultural society for a wide range of front line mental health workers, to be self reflexive and understand about different cultures' explanatory models for mental distress. It would create an awareness of patients' concerns, and would therefore be pertinent in training colleges for nurses, care workers and housing officers, and the police. It would support the government vision for seamless healthcare, and be useful for chaplains and religious leaders, both within hospitals and in the community.

Training would be of benefit to practitioners overseas aware of alternative theories of mental health causation; and students of medical anthropology and psychiatry. In today's world, it is not morally good enough that only academics and scholars are aware of plural models. Strategies to embed training as part of the core medical and health care education curriculum would reduce the need for optional add-on courses, for those post registration and in front-line mental healthcare practice.

Education for the Future

This book has contributed to our knowledge of existential, religious and spiritual elements of health, and these in turn enhanced our understanding of cultural interpretations of mental health conditions. If practitioner awareness of other frameworks of knowledge or cultural humility has alleviated just one person's suffering, this makes a difference to social well being. Certain principles of care and treatment from Pondicherry in India are transferable to UK minority ethnic populations, and would benefit the entire population.

In the new millennium, having collected data on health seeking strategies to address mental distress in India, and also undertaken research on mental health promotion strategies with migrant and refugee groups in UK, my over-riding goal was to raise awareness about cultural diversity issues with front line staff. I hoped that in some way enhanced awareness and humility at the front line would address not only the over-representation of black people under detention, but also the experiences of service users before, during, and after clinical care. To this end, I developed a series of training seminars which addressed that perceived need: to raise awareness of cultural BAME beliefs and knowledge about spirituality and health, and practitioner beliefs and values.

The topics I covered included: body and mind, spirit and soul, womanhood and conception, death and survival, mental health and religious experience. For some years I taught the material as optional courses in medical schools and universities, and for various health care trusts. I developed a strategy to honour cultural knowledge of minority ethnic groups, and improve relationships using enhanced therapeutic communication with professionals, to address social exclusion, and promote independence regarding pathways to access appropriate health care. It seemed obvious that if these seminars or others like them[144] were part of core training in medical and healthcare teaching organisations, this would address the need for 'sticking plaster' training amongst post registration staff. New training would focus on evidence based research of mental health promotion consultation with BAME service users, where their suggestions had been recorded, their needs listened to, and appropriate action taken. Training would go further than the one path of simply showing new migrants ways of accessing our health services.

In future it is important that training for staff is carried out concurrently with undergraduate student medical and allied health care workers, and with those already in post. Topics that might be additionally considered include the role of migration and religion, which could influence a person's well being regarding economic, political, or social disturbance. Research and consultation with BAME groups suggested it would be helpful to acknowledge the variety of migration histories, and hear narratives about reasons for migration.

Part of the training would acknowledge that ethnic minority groups are not homogenous: new migrants may bring conflicts from their country of origin. These may be conflicts of faith, religion, gender, class, and power. Then there are those who were born in Britain, and may have quite different expectations and ways of understanding the world, from their first generation parents and family. There may be wide cultural and moral differences between generations although their ethnicity and faith may be the same. Expectations of subsequent generations may be quite different from those of their forefathers.

It is critical we get education and training right: for current staff, medical, social care, health care, housing; and for trainees, as part of their core curriculum. It is important to ensure there is personal development for staff, so they become more aware of different strategies to address recovery alongside their clinical training. Courses would cover communication and negotiation strategies for dealing with patients whose frameworks of health are not concordant with practitioners.

If we want to influence policy decisions about cultural competencies, we need to lobby policy makers in UK, and government officials, to ensure The Mental Health Strategy bill is revised, in order to address ethnicity specifically, and not only as a small part of its equalities section. It would be useful to approach deans of education, to explore possibilities of having enhanced cultural competency / cultural humility training as part of their core curriculum.

A deeper collaboration would be ideal, so NHS psychiatrists have an accessible pathway to determine culturally appropriate care with their patients, so traditional and modern services can be used to access healing experts using different modalities. This might be like a Polyclinic, but with biomedical, complementary, alternative, and religious healing modalities available. Some

London boroughs already have something similar to this, but for end of life care. We also need it for mental health care.

It would be useful if the national government developed web based data for each NHS trust, where medical practitioners could access religious or alternative healing modalities relative to their patients' cultural requirements.

In these days of evidence based requirements, I feel it is essential for the government of the day to develop a central electronic archive, where all research reports (published or unpublished grey literature) are held and available. This would ensure that health strategies are evidence based on data from recommendations, and research is not duplicated.

In the USA, cultural competency is already required as an essential part of core mainstream medical education[145], [146]. In the UK, on-line training on the Equalities Act is an isolated individual training, which does not require direct self reflection or discussion with peers. However, within the UK's Education system, every school currently has a duty to illustrate ways they comply with the new government Equalities Act on Spiritual, Moral, Social and Cultural Well Being[147]. Schools undergo OFSTED inspections in these topics. I wonder why medical and health service educators are not asked to do the same. Perhaps it is a matter of time and public opinion.

When I began drafting this document cultural competency was the ideal: the acquiring of knowledge about this or that culture. This has been superseded by a new approach to global mental health: cultural humility. As well as focusing on a patient's clinical presentation we develop humility: to listen and to reflect; to appreciate cultural difference; to be aware of our own cultural values; and to negotiate appropriate treatment. I hope spiritual psychiatries continue to expand globally for the benefit of human kind.

APPENDICES
AND REFERENCES

UNDERSTANDING CONSCIOUSNESS

I tried to understand about Sri Aurobindo's concept of consciousness. I sought to work out what Sri Aurobindo's terms meant according to my own understanding, using Sat Prem's book on: 'Sri Aurobindo, or the adventures of consciousness, published in 1968, by the Sri Aurobindo Ashram Trust, in Pondicherry. The list provided below was created from my notes and quotes on the topic. I do not claim this is a definitive list, just my attempt to grasp concepts at the edge of my understanding.

See also:

http://www.aurobindo.ru/workings/satprem/adventure_of_consciousness_e.htm

The mind
  • Governs our will, and the action through thought or throat
  • One centre between the eyebrow, one at the throat
  • It is very slow, and likes routine and repetition

The Vital (Emotional level)
  • At the heart: governs our emotive being

- At the navel: governs power
- Between navel and genitals: governs negatives, anger and jealousy
- Aspiration: the key to mastery is silence
- Transparency allows us to pick up things
- Allows premonitions, but may allow negative entities

Illness

- Bacteria and viruses are agents: why do they affect one person and not another?
- Assumption: Allopathic medicine treats the symptoms and not the source
- If we can identify illness in the circumconscient layer, we can stop it
- Illness is also caused by a mismatch between levels

Circumconscient

- A layer around the body in which information can be seen or read

Subconscient / Subconscious

- This is the level of consciousness, as in an animal or plant
- Our past, immediate present, and remote past and future is held here
- It holds all the imprints of our present life, and all the imprints of our past lives
- The physical and subsconscient: At base of spine: governs physical and sexual being
- Assumption on Psycho-analysis: it fixes the mind on the unhealthy, rather than the divine. It suffuses the conscious mind with the unhealthy

The Physical

- the world is made of a single substance
- all terrestrial forms are made of the same stuff

- the history of earth is the slow conversion of force into consciousness into matter
- The body is a marvellous instrument: without the physical, divine life on earth is not possible
- We are in subjugation to the needs of the body in order to live, and through its organs to perceive the world

The Body
- Body is the point of insertion of consciousness into matter, and therefore one needs to work in the body.
- The body is an organ of light, which responds to the will of the mind, and can question the laws of nature
- Aim: towards transparency of person: to be like a receiving station for the divine
- The aim is to discover the principle of consciousness, which is the power to transform matter

Cosmic consciousness
- This is the universal consciousness that transcends the ego-centred individual and is in communion with the inner or subliminal dimension of the being.

The superconscient:
- Governs our thinking mind, spatially above our head. It links to higher supra-cognitive planes
- Beyond the brain, from which information may be channelled
- Other worlds populated by other beings, which exist outside of us. Beings that shape shift and can be seen according to our cultural specs.
- Transcendence, ecstasy

Supramental plane
- This lies above the higher mind, illumined mind, intuitive mind, and over-mind

- Within it one can see the past, the present, and the future
- The supramental consciousness sees everything. It can see from without and within. It links past, present, and future as one
- It carries the creative idea coeval with the executive force that builds the cosmos spontaneously and immaculately

Consciousness force
- *"a single current that circulates through us as it circulates through all things, and takes on one attribute or another, depending upon the particular level of its action"*.
- Awareness of it allows mastery over self, people and things…, i.e. it can act and transform matter
- This force can contact all matter, e.g. birds, plants, rocks, people
- Sound: can be used to raise consciousness: through use of mantras can manipulate life
- sat – chit- ananda: existence, consciousness, joy
- The force: the world traveller, explorer
- Matter is condensed energy

The psychic being
- which others call the 'soul'
- the link with what repeats, reincarnates
- The psychic grows between lives and during incarnations
- The experiences of the psychic form the psychic personality
- our individual centre
- it is eternal

At death
- the mental body, vital body, physical body all disintegrate
- Only the psychic remains, the others return to universal cosmos

Yogic state
- Consciousness freed from mental, vital, and physical turmoil
- Attachment: one may be as attached to renunciation as to possessions

The Chakras
- These are like receiving stations for different frequencies
- They are linked to different planes of consciousness

Spirits
- There are three spirits:
  - Psychic spirit (imminent)
  - Transcendent spirit (transcendent)
  - Cosmic spirit (universal)

The problem
- Materialists have not believed in the power of the spirit
- The spiritualists have not believed in the reality of matter
- We assume antennae create perception, rather than they were created in order to perceive.

Bridge during sleep
- We can be an agent of evolution of the earth
- We can sleep as a passive witness, or a spectator
- We need to integrate our consciousness of sleep to be masters of action
- By complete silence and immobility, the thread of an image will lead us on
- Or we can will to wake up once or twice a night, to remember
- We can learn to distinguish between ordinary dreams and experiences
- During sleep we can perceive the dead and other entities

- We can foresee the future, which already exists
- We can reach the Supramental plane

Aim in life
- To embrace all worldly activity and integrate the spiritual side
- To go to the divine, and bring the energies down into the physical, vital and mental
- To change the physical condition of humans, and control consciousness and ill health (that is the supramental aim)
- We need to embody high powers of consciousness: if we just obtain cosmic awareness it will do nothing for the earth
- Our aim is to harness divinity, and invite it to descend to terrestrial consciousness
- The secret: heaven and earth are equal. In matter: as above, so below

Exteriorisation
- *"Sleep, then, is a first tool; it can become conscious, increasingly conscious, ultimately reaching a point of development where we will become continuously conscious, whether on this side of the veil or the other.."*
- We can visit and see other planes of consciousness during sleep, deliberate OBE, and through continuous shifting while awake
- During sleep we are attached to a thread of the consciousness force, and we can perceive other worlds.
- Exteriorisation is equivalent to an out of body experience OBE
- We are living and acting on other planes simultaneously, all the time

SOUTH ASIAN EKTA MEETING IN HARROW

Over 60 people attended an EKTA meeting of the South Asian Service User group. Participants were Hindu, Jain, Christian and Muslim Asians, from India, Pakistan, and the Diaspora. The speaker from CNWL (*Central and North West London* NHS Foundation Trust), used a power point presentation to explain about CPA process (Care Programme Approach). The talk was translated into Gujarati and Hindi. One translator used the term 'medical model' to distinguish between that and other models (so often the underlying assumption was the medical model was the only model for considering health).

The EKTA group learnt CPA was an assessment to see whether or not mental health service users should get services, and what kind of services. A patient's Care Coordinator was supposed to put a care plan into action. One man in the audience suggested the CPA system was fine, but didn't actually happen. Other members of the audience responded:"*in practice funding doesn't come, and help doesn't come. It takes three or four months, and sometimes things are needed quickly*".

The speaker continued his power point talk. The CPA review was, he told us, held once a year, to find out what worked and what didn't work. It was a process, a series of meetings and relationships to identify a goal for the service user and to see what services were provided. It was important in building a relationship with service users: in principle patients could change their care coordinator. There needed to be trust and frequent contact between service users and staff, perhaps every three or six months. We were informed staff were measured on whether or not they made a copy of the CPA plan. If people felt they couldn't negotiate with their care coordinator, they could ask for an advocate or an interpreter, or ask a friend. This was considered to be part of the care plan.

During question time, one man mentioned for the second time that CPA did not happen. He said: "*most of what you are saying doesn't happen*". The speaker replied that the CPA was the ideal, and it should happen. The organiser said: "*you are showing such a good package, but we here assume this is not for us. We are identifying that it doesn't work, and there are barriers. There are barriers of relationship, trust, and bureaucracy, and there is no follow-up except in the form of letters*".

The EKTA organiser explained: "*most BAME communities favour oral communication, and prefer surgeries, so that they can talk with others, rather than receive written letters*". We were told that if there were complaints the PALS worker could help to draft a letter of complaint. More participants said they had not had any mention of CPA. The translator said the Care Coordinator was supposed to pull all strands of care together, and these included medical and social. However, the group explained that the response with them, the service users was always the same: "*you are on the waiting list*". They experienced little no follow-up.

People attending stood up and gave their personal testimonies. Person A had not had a care plan, but had a good psychiatrist, and was offered good medication. Person B had a CPA meeting where professionals did their paperwork, but they sent her different sheets to sign. One of the men attending the group said he was grateful as he had a crisis card with an emergency number to ring when he had problems. He said nobody should suffer in silence: "*In this community people do not insist they get the help that they need*".

The speaker emphasised patients needed to take control of their own care plan. He explained the CPA implementation group met monthly to discuss what worked, what didn't work, and to discuss themes people wanted to address in order to be safe. **The group were agreed that the presentation showed good practice, but stressed that it didn't happen in practice.** When Asian people were interviewed by their care coordinator, CPA was not mentioned. It was assumed, but not written down. One person claimed professionals used jargon and forgot clients didn't understand this jargon: "*You forget we don't understand the basic terms*". People with mental health problems were distressed, disempowered, and they didn't like to keep going forward.

It had been evident from the CNWL speaker's talk that staff in their offices, sitting behind desks, had developed an excellent package for supporting service users, but in fact, according to EKTA group participants, it didn't seem to have been put into practice in a way that ameliorated the experience of Asian mental health service users. It seemed systematic audit was required.

Part One Endnotes

1 Tobert 2001

2 Werneke 2009

3 Muskin 2000

4 Lake 2006, 2009

5 Stastny & Lehmann 2007

6 NSUN

7 CCHR 2010

8 Crossley 2006

9 Lake and Spiegel 2007

10 Safe Harbor

11 Mental Health Foundation

12 WHO

13 Tobert 2010

14 http://www.harrow.gov.uk/info/200088/statistics_and_census_information/496/census_2011-detailed_results_and_reports

15 Time to Change EKTA, 2011

16 In London, Wolfson, UCL, Rcpsych

17 E.g. Durham, Kent, Brunel

18 Transcultural Psychiatry SIG

19 Count Me in 2010

20 Delivering Race Equality 2005

21 RAWOrg 2011

22 Race for Health

23 BME NHS Network

24 http://www.communitycare.co.uk/Articles/2009/11/25/113253/mental-health-act-detentions-rise-sharply-for-bme-groups.htm

25 http://www.youngminds.org.uk/mailshot-news/group-urges-data-on-bme-mental-health-to-be-published

26 http://warwick.academia.edu/SwaranSingh/Papers/447687/Ethnicity_and_Detention_Under_the_Mental_Health_Act

27 http://www.guardian.co.uk/society/joepublic/2011/mar/01/race-equality-mental-health

[28] Alan Sanderson, http://www.spiritrelease.com/sandersonprofile.htm

[29] Andrew Powell, http://www.rcpsych.ac.uk/college/specialinterestgroups/spirituality/

[30] Dinesh Bhugra, http://www.iop.kcl.ac.uk/departments/?locator=396

[31] Kamaldeep Bhui. 2007

[32] Dein S, 2001, 2005, 2008

[33] Malidoma Some 1994

[34] Kharitidi 1995

[35] Clarke 2010

[36] Spiritual Crisis Network

[37] psychosisspirituality@yahoogroups.com

[38] Fuller 2004

[39] Parry 1994

Part Two Endnotes

[40] Basu 2000

[41] Miovic 2010

[42] Miovic 2004

[43] Shaik Hasan Sahib Qadhiri 1998

[44] BMA News 2003, 1

[45] Census of India 1961

[46] Kesav 2001; 30

[47] Sivamayan 2000

[48] Packirisamy 2000

[49] Census of India 1961

[50] Packirisamy 2000

[51] Irudayam 1999

[52] Ibid; 24

[53] Ibid; 28

Part Three Endnotes

[54] Eisenbruch 1984

[55] Canault 1998

[56] Dr Basu, Integral Health 2000

[57] Joshi et al 2008

[58] Clarke 2010

[59] Tobert 2005

[60] Dein 2008

[61] Clarke 2010

[62] Grof 1989

[63] Tobert 2000

Part Four Endnotes

[64] Mistry D 2002

[65] Shree Gurudev, Katkar S

[66] Varma S 2010

[67] Transpersonal Psychology UK

[68] Kakar 1991

[69] Varma, S 2005

[70] Joel et al, Indian Journal of Psychiatry 2006

[71] Saravanan et al 2008

[72] Woo-kyoung et al 2009

[73] Germer 2009

[74] Koenig 2007

[75] Dept Health 2009

[76] Woodhouse 1996

[77] Good 1994

[78] Reichel-Dolmatoff 1997

[79] Manning Upstream Healthcare

[80] Argyris 1990

[81] Bellinger 2004

[82] Tobert 2010b

[83] CNWL http://www.cnwl.nhs.uk/services/community-recovery/recovery-college/

[84] NSUN: *www.nsun.org.uk/*

[85] Testimony Project: http://www.webarchive.org.uk/ukwa/target/66158832/

[86] http://www.bl.uk/reshelp/findhelprestype/sound/ohist/ohcoll/ohhealth/health.html

[87] CCHR, Compendium, 1969

[88] Levin 2001

[89] Race For Health 2011

[90] http://www.uhsm.nhs.uk/research/Pages/abcgroup.aspx

[91] Tobert 2010 a & b

[92] Tobert 2010 a & b

[93] Harvey 2003

[94] Kübler-Ross 1970

[95] Basu 2000

[96] NAMAH, Journal of New Approaches to Medicine & Health

[97] Miovic 2010

[98] Miovic 2009

[99] http://www.dosseydossey.com/larry/default.html, Dossey, *Recovering the Soul* (*1989*)

[100] Tobert 2010 a and b

[101] Black, Asian, and Minority Ethnic groups

Part Five Endnotes

[102] Office for National Statistics.

[103] Neighbourhood.statistics.gov.uk.

[104] OFSTED, Office for Standards in Education, Children's Services and Skills: report directly to Parliament

[105] Care Quality Commission 2011

[106] Care Quality Commission 2011, p.18

[107] Argyris 1983

[108] Diverse Minds 1997, http://www.mind.org.uk/diverseminds

[109] Fernando 2003

[110] http://www.psychminded.co.uk/

[111] Page 2011

[112] When a meeting, or part thereof, is held under the **Chatham House Rule**, participants are free to use the information received, but neither the identity nor the affiliation of the speaker(s), nor that of any other participant, may be revealed.

[113] AMHP: *approved mental health professional*

[114] http://www.dineshbhugra.net/

[115] Cornelison et al 2011

[116] For UK based transcultural psychiatry:

http://www.wolfson.qmul.ac.uk/psychiatry/

http://www.ucl.ac.uk/slms/

http://transculturalpsychiatry.gla.ac.uk/

http://www.rcpsych.ac.uk/workinpsychiatry/specialinterestgroups/transculturalpsychiatry.aspx

[117] Dein et al 2008, Tobert 2010a, b,

[118] Cornelissen 2012

[119] Passi V (ed) 2011

[120] Equality and Human Rights Commission 2012

[121] Tobert 2010a

[122] Tobert 2010b

[123] Mind in Harrow

[124] CNWL

[125] Hornstein 2009

[126] Moncrieff 2010

[127] Watters 2011

[128] Stastny & Lehmann 2007

[129] Testimony Project

[130] Bridging Cultures: http://www.aethos.org.uk/research

[131] EKTA Reaching the South Asian community in Harrow, Time to Change pilot project, 2011

[132] CNWL http://www.cnwl.nhs.uk/recovery-college/

[133] Singh et al 2013

[134] Minority Ethnic Health. List aimed at professionals who strive to improve health of minority ethnic communities in UK

[135] Bhui http://bjp.rcpsych.org/content/178/6/575.2

[136] Kleinman 1988

[137] Bhui and Bhugra 2002

[138] Clements H 1957

[139] Royal College of Psychiatrists, http://rcpsych.ac.uk/pdf/PS03_2011.pdf

[140] Manning C: http://www.upstreamhealthcare.org/upstream.html

[141] Turner V 1968

[142] http://www.dineshbhugra.net/dbhindicinema.html

[143] British Holistic Medical Association www.bhma.org/ *and* Scientific and Medical Network https://www.scimednet.org

[144] EHI Conferences

[145] Kripalani, Bussey-Jones, Katz, et al, 2006

[146] https://psych.ucsf.edu/sfgh/chtf/

[147] Equality Act 2010: 1

REFERENCES AND RESOURCES

Afiya Trust, www.afiya-trust.org/

Argyris C 1990, Overcoming Organizational Defenses, Facilitating Organizational Learning, Boston. http://www.systems-thinking.org/loi/loi.htm

Argyris, C 1983, Action Science and Intervention, Applied Behavioural Science, vol.19. 2 http://jab.sagepub.com/content/19/2/115.abstract

Barker, P Buchanan-Barker P (eds) 2003, Spirituality and Mental Health: Breakthrough, Whurr, 1-86156-392-2,

Basu, S. 2000, Integral Health, SAIIIHR, Pondicherry, India

Bellinger G 2004, http://www.systems-thinking.org/loi/loi.htm

Bentall RP: 2003*Madness Explained: Psychosis and Human Nature.* London: Penguin

Bhui K and Bhugra D, 2002. Explanatory models for mental distress: implications for clinical practice and research, British Journal of Psychiatry

Bhui K, et al. 2007 – Culture and Mental Health: A Comprehensive Textbook

Bhui K 2001, Over-representation of Black people in secure psychiatric facilities http://bjp.rcpsych.org/content/178/6/575.2

BMA News 2003, 1, http://bma.org.uk

BME NHS Network, http://www.nationalnhsbmenetwork.org.uk/site/ , http://www.nhsbmenetwork.org.uk/

Bhugra D, http://www.iop.kcl.ac.uk/departments/?locator=396

Bhugra, D, http://www.dineshbhugra.net/

British Library, http://www.bl.uk/reshelp/findhelprestype/sound/ohist/ohcoll/ohhealth/health.html

Canault, N. 1998 Comment paye-t-on la faute de nos ancetres, Desclee deBrouwer, Pari

Cant S, Sharma U 1999, A New Medical Pluralism: Complementary Medicine, Doctors, Patients and the State

Care Quality Commission, 2011, Monitoring the Mental Health Act in 2010/11, http://www.cqc.org.uk/sites/default/files/media/documents/cqc_mha_report_2011_main_final.pdf

CCHR, Psychiatry: The Compendium, http://www.cchr.co.uk/

Census of India 1961 (publ 1966), Vol 9, Madras, part XI D, Temples, Vol.2 & 6, (IS 433/2

Chatham House Rule: http://www.chathamhouse.org.uk/about/chathamhouserule/

Chuengsatiansup K, 2003, Spirituality and health: an initial proposal to incorporate spiritual health in health impact assessment, Environmental Impact Assessment Review, Elsevier, Volume 23, Issue 1, 3–15

Clarke I (ed.), 2010 Psychosis and Spirituality: Exploring the New Frontier, Wiley Publishers,

Claus, P, 1984, Medical Anthropology And The Ethnography Of Spirit Possession, California State University East Bay, Hayward, CA., U.S.A.

Clements H, 1957, Headaches and Migraine, Health for All Publishing, Surrey

CNWL 2010, http://www.cnwl.nhs.uk/ Faith and Spirituality in Patient Care

CNWL2012http://www.cnwl.nhs.uk/services/community-recovery/recovery-college

CommunityCare:http://www.communitycare.co.uk/Articles/2009/11/25/113253/mental-health-act-detentions-rise-sharply-for-bme-groups.htm

Cornelissen, M., Misra, G. & Varma S. (Eds.) 2011, *Foundations of Indian Psychology: Concepts and Theories*, Vol. I. New Delhi: Pearson.

Cornelissen Matthijs 2012, Types of knowledge and what they allow us to see. How our research methods affect the quality of our psychological understanding. http://www.ipi.org.in/texts/matthijs/mc-tok-ppb.php

Count Me in 2010, Care Quality Commission, London http://www.cqc.org.uk/guidanceforprofessionals/mentalhealth/countmeincensus/countmeincensus2010.cfm

Critical Psychiatry: http://www.critpsynet.freeuk.com/critpsynet.htm http://www.criticalpsychiatry.co.uk/

Crossley, N, 2006, *Contesting Psychiatry*, Routledge

Dein S, 2001, The Use of Traditional Healing in South Asian Psychiatric Patients in the U.K, Transcultural Psychiatry vol. 38 no. 2 243-257

Dein 2005, Spirituality and treatment choices by South and East Asian women with serious mental illness. Transcultural Psychiatry, 2005 42: 630-656

Dein, S 2008, Jinn, Psychiatry and Contested Notions of Misfortune among East London Bangladeshis Transcultural Psychiatry March 1, 2008 45: 31-55

Delivering Race Equality report 2005, http://www.dh.gov.uk/en/Publicationsandstatistics/Publications/PublicationsPolicyAnd Guidance/DH_4100773

Department of Health 2009, Guidelines on Religion and Faith for Mental Health

Diverse Minds 1997, http://www.mind.org.uk/diverseminds

Dossey, *L 1989,* Recovering the Soul, Bantam Books http://www.dosseydossey.com/larry/default.html,

EHI Conferences, Ethnic Health Initiative *www.bmehealth.org/*

Eisenbruch M, 1984, Cross-cultural aspects of bereavement. I: A conceptual framework for comparative analysis. Culture, Medicine and Psychiatry, 8, 283-309.

EKTA, Reaching the South Asian Community, Time To Change, 2011 http://www.time-to-change.org.uk/blog/harrow-beacon-hope

Equality and Human Rights Commission 2012, Research report 84: Religion or belief, equality and human rights in England and Wales

EqualityAct2010,https://www.gov.uk/equality-act-2010-guidance

Fernando, S 2003, Cultural diversity, mental health and psychiatry: the struggle against racism, Routledge

Fuller, C J 2004, *The Camphor Flame:* Popular Hinduism and Society in India, Princeton University Press, 069112048X,

Germer, C. 2009, The Mindful Path to Self-compassion, Guildford Press

Good B. J 1994 – *Medicine, Rationality, and Experience:* An Anthropological Perspective (Lewis Henry Morgan Lecture Series.)

Grof, S & C 1989, Spiritual Emergency: When Personal Transformation Becomes a Crisis (New Consciousness Readers), Penguin Putnam

Guardian: http://www.guardian.co.uk/society/joepublic/2011/mar/01/race-equality-mental-health

Harvey G, 2003.Shamanism: a reader, Routledge,

Helman C, 2007, Culture, Health and Illness, Hodder Arnold

Hornstein, G, 2009, Agnes's Jacket: a psychologist's search for the meaning of madness, Rodale books

Irudayam 1999, Vailankanni Cathedral

Kleinman A, 1988, Rethinking Psychiatry: from Cultural Category to Personal Experience. New York: Free Press

Kleinman A, Eisenberg L, Good B 1978, Culture, Illness, and Care, Annals of Internal Medicine, vol. 88 (2) 251-258

Koenig, H. G. 2007 Spirituality in Patient Care, Templeton Foundation Press

Kripalani, Bussey-Jones, Katz, et al, 2006, , A Prescription for Cultural Competence in Medical Education, J Gen Intern Med; 21(10): 1116–1120 http://www.ncbi.nlm.nih.gov/pmc/articles/PMC1831630/

Kübler-Ross, E 1970, On death and Dying, Routledge

Jadhav, S *2004,* How culture bound is 'cultural' psychiatry? Bulletin of International Psychiatry of the Royal College of Psychiatrists, http://www.indianpsychiatry.com

Joel D, Sathyaseelan M, Jayakaran R, Vijayakumar C, Muthurathnam S and Jacob K.S. 2006, A biomedical educational intervention to change explanatory models of psychosis among community health workers in South India, Indian J Psychiatry, 48(3):138–142.

Joshi et al 2008, Gujarati Elders, Mind in Harrow & UCLAN

Kakar, S 1991 Shamans, Mystics, and Doctors, University of Chicago Press,

Katkar, S, http://shreevidyamahayog.org/Inner/Home.aspx

Kharitidi, O 1995, Entering the Circle, Harper One

Kübler-Ross E, 1970, On Death and Dying, Simon & Schuster/ Touchstone

Lake, J 2009, *Integrative mental health care:* therapist's handbook, Norton & Co.

Lake J, Spiegel D, 2007, *Complementary and Alternative Treatments in Mental Health Care*, American Psychiatric Pub

Lake J, 2006, *Textbook of Integrative Mental Health Care,* Thieme,

Levin J 2001, God, Faith, and Health: Exploring the Spirituality-Healing Connection

Wiley and Sons

Malidoma Some, 1994, Of water and the Spirit, Compass

Manning C http://www.upstreamhealthcare.org/upstream.html

Mental Health Foundation, Doing Research Ourselves, 2001, http://www.mentalhealth.org.uk/publications/

Minority Ethnic Health email list: *www.jiscmail.ac.uk/lists/minority-ethnic-health.html*

Miovic, M 2010, Sri Aurobindo and Transpersonal Psychology, http://www.sciy.org/2010/01/02/sri-aurobindo-and-transpersonal-psychology-by-michael-miovic-md/

Miovic M 2009, The relevance of non-local studies to health, NAMAH, Vol 17; no.3

Miovic, M. 2004, "An Introduction to Spiritual Psychology: Overview of the Literature, East and West," Harvard Review of Psychiatry, vol 12 (2), pp. 1-11.

Mistry, D 2002, http://meherhomoeopath.com/clinicalRecorder.aspx , http://www.njhonline.com/abstract/homeo_clinical_case_recorder4.shtml

Moncrieff J 2010, Psychiatric diagnosis as a political device. *Soc Theor Health*, 8(4), 370

Muskin, P, (ed) 2000, *Complementary and alternative medicine and psychiatry*, Volume 19, Issue 1, American Psychiatric Press.

NAMAH, Journal of New Approaches to Medicine & Health, http://www.namahjournal.com/

Neighbourhood.statistics.gov.uk

NSMFH, National Spirituality and Mental Health Forum http://mhspirituality.org.uk/

NSUN, National Service User Group, http://www.nsun.org.uk/

NSUN, http://www.nsun.org.uk/get-involved/survivor_involvement/

Office for National Statistics. http://www.statistics.gov.uk http://www.ons.gov.uk/ons/rel/census/2011-census/key-statistics-for-local-authorities-in-england-and-wales/sty-non-uk-born-population.html

OFSTED, Office for Standards in Education http://www.ofsted.gov.uk/

Packirisamy G 2000, Ramanathaswamy Temple, A Guide Book of Rameswaram Dhanushkodi

Page R 2011, Reverse Commissioning Success, http://www.nhsbmenetwork.org.uk/

Parry, J. 1994, Death in Banaras, Cambridge University Press

Passi V (ed) 2011, *Excellence in Medical Education*, *AOME, 1*

Powell A, http://www.rcpsych.ac.uk/college/specialinterestgroups/spirituality/

Psychiatry: *The* Compendium, CCHR, *Citizens Commission on Human Rights*

Psychminded: http://www.psychminded.co.uk/

Psychosis and Spirituality psychosisspirituality@yahoogroups.com

Race for Health, http://www.raceforhealth.org/

Race for Health 2011, Tackling Health Inequalities in the New NHS

Raguram, R, Venkateswaran A, Ramakrishna J 2002, Traditional community resources for mental health: temple healing from India, *British Medical Journal*;325:38-40.

Race for Health, http://www.raceforhealth.org/

RAWOrg 2011, The End of Delivering Race Equality? http://www.mind.org.uk/news/5030_delivering_race_equality_did_not_fully_deliver_claims_thinktank

Reichel-Dolmatoff *G 1997* Rainforest Shamans: Tukano Indians of the Northwest Amazon, Totnes, Foxhole, UK

Royal College of Psychiatrists: http://rcpsych.ac.uk/pdf/PS03_2011.pdf Recommendations for psychiatrists on spirituality and religion, Position Statement PS03/2011

Safe Harbor web site, http://www.alternativementalhealth.com/

Sanderson A, http://www.spiritrelease.com/sandersonprofile.htm

Saravanan B, Jacob KS, Deepak MG, Prince M, David AS, Bhugra D. 2008, Perceptions about psychosis and psychiatric services: a qualitative study from Vellore, India., Soc Psychiatry Psychiatr Epidemiol. 43(3):231-8

Satprem 1993, Adventures in Consciousness, Institute for Evolutionary Research, New York

Shaik Hasan Sahib Qadhiri 1998, Nagore Mosque

Shree Gurudev Shrivas Katkar http://shreevidyamahayog.org/Inner/AboutShreeGurudev.aspx

Singh S P, Burns T, Tyrer P, Islam Z, Parsons H and Crawford M J , 2013. Ethnicity as a predictor of detention under the Mental Health Act, Psychological Medicine, CUP, 24.06.13

Sivamayam 2000, Navagraha Temple, Suriyanarkoil, Guide Book

Some, Malidoma 1994, Of Water and the Spirit, Compass

Spiritual Crisis Network, http://www.spiritualcrisisnetwork.org.uk/

Sri Aurobindo Ashram, http://www.sriaurobindoashram.org/

Sri Ramana Marshi Ashram, http://www.sriramanamaharshi.org/

Stastny P, Lehmann P, (eds) 2007, *Alternatives Beyond Psychiatry*, Peter Lehmann Publishing

Szasz TS, 1974, *The Myth of Mental Illness.* New York: Harper and Row

Testimony Project 2000 http://www.insidestories.org/

Time to Change http://www.time-to-change.org.uk/

Tobert N. 2000, *Anegondi: Architectural Ethnography of a Royal Village in India,* Vijayanagara Research Monograph, no.7, Manohar Press, New Delhi

Tobert N 2001a, Psychiatrists and Shamans: a comparison, in NAMAH (New Approaches to Medicine and Health), vol. 8, no. 2, SAHIIIR, Pondicherry, India

Tobert, N. 2001b, Consciousness and Health: another perspective from India, Network: Scientific and Medical Network Review, no. 75

Tobert, N 2007, In-Sanity: Explanatory Models for Religious Experience, Occasional Paper no.3, Series 3, Religious Experience Research Centre, University of Wales, Lampeter

Tobert N, 2008 Mental Health Needs Assessment with BME Communities, NHS Harrow

Tobert N, 2010a Bridging Cultures, Dissolving Barriers, Mental Health Promotion With BME Communities, End of Year Evaluation Report 2009 / 2010, NHS Harrow

Tobert N 2010b, Somali Advocacy Final Report Harrow, Kings Fund

Tobert N 2013, Cultural Equalities, Training Resource Pack for Medical, Health and Social Care

Transpersonal Psychology UK http://www.transpersonalcentre. co.uk/, http://www.northampton.ac.uk/courses/286/transpersonal-psychology-and-consciousness-studies-msc/ , http://www.ljmu.ac.uk/ NSP/CTP.htm, http://www.transpersonalacademy.co.uk/

Transcultural Psychiatry SIG Royal College of Psychiatry http:// www.rcpsych.ac.uk/rollofhonour/specialinterestgroups/ transculturalpsychiatry/ http://www.rcpsych.ac.uk/workinpsychiatry/ specialinterestgroups/transculturalpsychiatry.aspx

Transcultural psychiatry courses:
http://www.wolfson.qmul.ac.uk/psychiatry/
http://www.ucl.ac.uk/slms/
http://transculturalpsychiatry.gla.ac.uk/

Tukelocklingam K. 1961 (publ 1966), Census of India Vol 9, Tamil Nadu, part XI D, Temples, Vol. VII (1), Tanjur

Turner, Victor. [1968] 1981 reprint. *The Drums of Affliction: A Study of Religious Processes Among the Ndembu of Zambia.* Ithaca, NY:

Varma, S 2010 http://www.herenow4u.net/index.php?id=76116

Varma, S. (2005). From the self to the Self: An exposition on personality based on the works of Sri Aurobindo. In K.R. Rao & S.M. Bhatt (Eds.), Towards a Spiritual psychology New Delhi: Samvad.

Watters E 2011, Crazy Like Us: Globalization of the American Psyche, Barnes & Noble

Werneke U, 2009, CPD module on Complementary and Alternative approaches: http://www.psychiatrycpd.co.uk/learningmodules/

WHO report 2010, http://www.who.int/mental_health/policy/mhtargeting/en/index.html

WHO Library Promoting mental health: 2005 www.who.int/bulletin/bulletin_board/83/ustun11051

WHO 1996, Constitution of the World Health Organisation

Woo-kyoung A, Proctor C and Flanagan E, 2009, Mental Health Clinicians' Beliefs About the Biological, Psychological, and Environmental Bases of Mental Disorders, Cogn Sci. 2009 March; 33 (2)

Woodhouse, M, *1996 Paradigm Wars*: Worldviews for a New Age

World Health Organisation, http://www.euro.who.int/en/home

Young Minds http://www.youngminds.org.uk/news/news

ABOUT THE AUTHOR

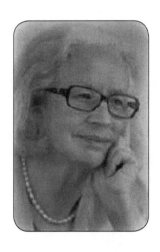

Dr Natalie Tobert is a British medical anthropologist, who has undertaken research in India, United Kingdom, and the Sudan. Her interests, which include health promotion among minority groups, explore the crossroads between cultural understanding, religious experience, and mental wellbeing. They have inspired *Spiritual Psychiatries*, an exploration of Indian mental health traditions and their relevance for global multicultural populations.

She has taught seminars in mental health equality and cultural diversity at universities, medical schools, hospitals, and religious institutions throughout the UK. She is currently the education director at Aethos Consultancy, and has facilitated workshops in Sweden, and Switzerland.

Printed in Great Britain
by Amazon.co.uk, Ltd.,
Marston Gate.